Skilled Hands

Skilled Hands

SURGERY AT

The University of Texas Medical School at Houston

William Henry Kellar

Heather Green Wooten

ISBN: 978-0-9846070-1-3

In memory of

James H. “Red” Duke, M.D.

CONTENTS

ILLUSTRATIONS

All photos courtesy: Department of Surgery, The University of Texas Medical School at Houston.

FOREWORD

On the 30th anniversary of The University of Texas Medical School at Houston (UTHealth Medical School) in the fall of 2000, I had the opportunity to publish a 30-year history of this very special medical school located in the heart of Houston's Texas Medical Center. This medical school is one of six professional schools comprising The University of Texas Health Science Center at Houston (UTHealth). Much has changed over the years since Gov. Preston Smith came to Houston on June 13,1969 to sign enabling legislation to launch UT's newest medical school at the time.

That same year a new dean, Cheves McCord Smythe, M.D., arrived in Houston to take the helm and build the school from the ground up. Harvard educated and Charleston savvy, Smythe had no faculty, no buildings, and no students. What he did have was an experienced vision and a mandate to move quickly.

High on his list was to find a chairman for surgery who was young yet accomplished, highly skilled at his craft and a team player determined to build an academic surgical department that would serve the needs of this community while growing the reputation and the reach of the new medical school and its primary hospital affiliate, Hermann Hospital (today Memorial Herman Hospital - Texas Medical Center).

Smythe found that surgeon/leader at the University of Pennsylvania in Dr. Stanley Dudrick. Dudrick launched the department around his own pioneering interests in nutritional research and in 1972 reached to Afghanastan to find a young surgical talent named Dr. James H. "Red" Duke, Jr. Duke would join Dr. Ted Copeland, a highly decorated Viet Nam surgeon who shared a similar interest in academic medicine, nutrition, and surgery. As the book you hold will tell, that small cadre of three full-time faculty got busy and showed what hard work and creativity could yield. Along the way they demonstrated interdisciplinary and interinstitutional teamwork working with basic scientists and clinicians throughout the school and medical community.

Stanley Dudrick was followed as chair by Dr. Frank Moody who arrived from The University of Utah in 1982. The department's current chairman, Dr. Richard Andrassy came from San Antonio in 1985 and followed Moody in the leadership role a decade later. Andrassy continues to build and shape the department in ways never dreamed of back in the early 1970s with the admiration of both former chairman whom I've visited with in recent months.

William Henry Kellar and Heather Green Wooten have done an outstanding job telling the department's story from the earliest days to the present. This is the story of what three surgical chairs and a long list of talented faculty, surgeons in training, and staff can accomplish building a program that advances our knowledge and expertise to the bedside—saving countless lives on a daily basis while training the next generation of surgeons. Today, UTHealth Medical School's Department of Surgery takes its place amongst the finest in the nation.

Successful programs don't happen by accident. It all starts with leadership and commitment by those in charge. Perhaps General George S. Patton said it best when he outlined his own philosophy for building a program of excellence. Dudrick, Moody, and Andrassy all seem to have been on same page with Patton who said, "Don't tell people how to do things, tell them what to do and let them surprise you with their results."

From Memorial Herman Hospital's Life Flight visible in the Houston area skies 24/7 to advanced laparoscopic surgery and robotics, this Department of Surgery has had a major hand—a skilled hand—in rewriting the history of surgery as we know it. The product of their efforts has been much more than patient outcomes and advancements in surgical practice, it also translates into the human currency of training outstanding surgeons who are increasingly leading programs around the country and beyond.

While in 2000 I told the story of the UT Medical School at large through conversations with the deans who came here to build it, this is a book that takes you inside the institution to the departmental level to see how talented people given outstanding leadership and opportunities continue to surprise through their creativity and results. They are but one department of nearly two dozen comprising this medical school but as surgeons do so well, they cut to the chase and shine a bright operating light on the true value of academic medicine in the grand scheme of American medicine.

Bryant Boutwell, Dr.P.H.
John P. McGovern Professor of Oslerian Medicine
Distinguished Teaching Professor
Author, *Conversation with a Medical School* (1999)

PREFACE AND ACKNOWLEDGMENTS

Surgery—the term itself carries so many connotations, and in many, it engenders conflicting emotions ranging from fear and despair to confidence and hope. In reading the history of how surgery evolved and developed over time, one finds stories both macabre and miraculous. Evidence suggests that ancient Egyptians practiced surgery, and their burial and mummification practices certainly offered opportunities to learn something of human anatomy.

During the Roman era, around 157 A.D., scholars point to Galen, who was a "physician to the gladiators" and referred to as "one of the first trauma surgeons" due to his role in setting broken bones, amputating limbs, and otherwise tending to the battle wounds of his charges. When he interviewed for the post, he rather colorfully demonstrated his ability by bringing with him a monkey, cutting open its stomach, and then sewing it back together again. He was said to have asked, "Can anyone else do that?" He got the job, and the monkey survived the interview, too.[1]

In North America, most likely in what today is the state of Texas, the Spanish explorer Alvar Nuñez Cabeza de Vaca is acknowledged to have been a European pioneer of surgery in the New World when in 1535, he removed an arrow from the chest of a Native American and sewed the incision with thread made of deer hide. The patient survived, and so did de Vaca.[2]

By contrast, today's modern surgeons work in spotlessly clean, highly sanitized operating rooms often using minimally invasive procedures, robots, and all of the latest in anesthesia and surgical technology. Interestingly, much of this great leap forward in surgical practice occurred during the past fifty years, an amazing example of change over time.

Thus, when Dr. Richard J. Andrassy, Chairman of the Department of Surgery at The University of Texas Medical School at Houston, contacted me about writing a history of the department, I jumped at the chance. Over the years, I have written several books about Houston's medical history and the institutions of the Texas Medical Center. In the course of my research for these projects I interviewed many physicians and many surgeons. I found that most surgeons chose their specialty primarily because they wanted to "fix" people whose bodies were broken or damaged in some way. They were supremely confident in their ability, courageous in their willingness to employ drastic measures, and took great satisfaction in being able to affect an immediate and noticeable repair for their patients. The prospect of learning more about this most dramatic of medical specialties and writing about some of these remarkable people and their incredible skills presented both a challenge and an incredible opportunity that I embraced immediately.

As I began to work on this project, I contacted medical historian Heather Green Wooten, PhD, and engaged her to help as a coauthor. Wooten is the author of two excellent books on Texas medical history, *The Polio Years in Texas: Battling a Terrifying Unknown* (Texas A&M University Press, 2009); and *Old Red: Pioneering Medical Education in Texas* (Texas State Historical Association, 2012), both of which introduced her to many of the sources and archives in which we would work for this project. In addition to conducting new research specifically for this project, we were able to draw upon some of our previous work that helped provide context for this study. I conducted a series of oral history interviews, while Heather mined the collections at local archives. Together, we assembled our notes and photocopies from both primary and secondary sources found in the collections of the Houston Metropolitan Research Center of the Houston Public Library, the John P. McGovern Historical Collections and Research Center of the Texas Medical Center Library, Special Collections of the University of Houston–Clear Lake Alfred R. Neumann Library, materials provided by The University of Texas Medical School at Houston Department of Surgery, and various websites on the Internet. Sources are cited in the endnotes with each chapter, and oral history interviewees are listed in the "Note on Sources" at the end of this book. This study, then, is based upon a series of oral history interviews and on a variety of primary and secondary sources.

The final book, *Skilled Hands: Surgery at The University of Texas Medical School at Houston,* is comprised of ten chapters, including an epilogue, beginning in chapter one with the decision by the state legislature in 1969 to authorize creation of a new University of Texas Medical School in Houston. The first chapter explores the question of how one begins to build a medical school from scratch, the monumental task that fell to the founding dean, Dr. Cheves McCord Smythe. Chapter two documents the challenge of creating a new academic department of surgery: recruiting the founding chairman, Dr. Stanley J. Dudrick, along with his initial faculty and students; and the issues related to establishing relations with the primary teaching hospital, Hermann Hospital. Chapter three looks at the early growth of the department during the 1970s, including the innovative development of the Life Flight helicopter ambulance service in conjunction with Hermann Hospital. Chapter four is an overview of the department's key role in organ transplantation and in FDA trials of immunosuppressant drugs, key to the success of organ transplantation today. Chapter five examines how the department continued to grow and mature under the leadership of its second chairman, Dr. Frank G. Moody. Chapter six introduces the third department chairman, Dr. Richard J. Andrassy, and explores some of the changes in pediatric surgery over time. The remaining chapters focus on changes in trauma and acute care surgery (chapter seven); the continuing evolution of the department (chapter eight); the formation of new surgical departments (chapter nine); and an epilogue that examines the concept of change over time as it relates to surgery and the Department of Surgery at the Medical School.

Skilled Hands offers a unique perspective primarily from the point of view of those who first established The University of Texas Medical School in Houston and from many of those who served as faculty, residents, and students in the Department of Surgery during its forty-plus years of history. This work helps to fill a gap in the existing literature of the history of the Medical School and its increasingly prominent place in academic medicine and as one of the major institutions of the Texas Medical Center. It will also be useful to anyone with an interest in the history of The University of Texas Medical School at Houston and the role of its Department of Surgery, as it grew from a mere notion of the state legislature to become the sixth-largest medical school in the country. Furthermore, the book also provides fascinating insight into the evolution of surgical practices within the field through the eyes of those who made and implemented such changes.

This book would not have been possible without the support of Richard J. Andrassy, MD, Professor and Chairman of the Department of Surgery, whose deep appreciation for history inspired him to commit fully to the project. Along with this, we also would like to thank Dr. Giuseppe N. Colasurdo, President of The University of Texas Health Science Center at Houston (UTHealth) and Dean of the Medical School, for his continued support of the Department of Surgery. There are many others who made substantial contributions to this project, including many current and former faculty who participated in the oral history interviews. Their names and the dates of their interviews appear in the "Note on Sources." In addition, we would like to acknowledge former deans of the Medical School, Drs. Cheves M. Smythe and John C. Ribble; Drs. Denton A. Cooley and O. H. "Bud" Frazier of the Texas Heart Institute; Dr. Kenneth L. Mattox, Baylor College of Medicine; and author Dr. Bryant Boutwell, UTHealth; all of whom graciously made time in their busy schedules to be interviewed for this project. Several alumni of the Department of Surgery kindly shared their reminiscences, including: Drs. Christopher W. Conner, Timothy A. Dernbach, James Flynn, Richard Hofstetter, Greg R. Pahnke, Ming Pan, Benjamin S. Paulson, Eric K. Peden, Johnny Perez, Debra A. Reilly, and George Van Buren II. Administrative assistance for the project came from the unfailingly pleasant Elizabeth "Mickey" Clouser, Senior Executive Assistant to Richard J. Andrassy, MD, Professor and Chairman, Department of Surgery. On the business side of the project, we are grateful to Cynthia Huehlefeld, Director of Management Operations and her successor, Patricia Birkmeyer at UTHealth. Additionally, Suzanne Mascola ably transcribed the oral history interviews, and historian Elisabeth O'Kane Lipartito read and commented on the manuscript, offering numerous suggestions that helped to improve the final draft. We also wish to express our gratitude to Philip Montgomery and Alethea Drexler of the John P. McGovern Historical Collections and Research Center, Texas Medical Center Library, whose knowledge of the center's vast collections is unsurpassed and proved to be exceedingly helpful in our research. Finally, to the many others without whose help this project could not have been accomplished, our deepest and most sincere thanks.

—William Henry Kellar and Heather Green Wooten

Introduction

"I think your solution is just. But why think?
Why not try the experiment?"
John Hunter to Edward Jenner, August 2, 1775.

The workings of the human body have captivated mankind's attention for centuries. Ever since ancient Greek physicians began probing the human interior, anatomists and surgeons have painstakingly unlocked many secrets relative to bodily structure and function, while others remain a mystery. The rationale behind anatomic research is simple: to know the body is to discover legitimate means of healing it. The role of the surgeon is to incorporate available medical knowledge with the process of opening up individuals in order to cure them. Historically, the act of cutting into a living person was brutal and involved great risk, especially prior to the development of anesthetics or antiseptics. The benefits of surgery, while always apparent to some degree, have risen substantially only with the scientific and clinical advancement of the practice. When The University of Texas Medical School at Houston welcomed its first class of students in 1972, professors within the newly created Department of Surgery possessed a firm professional foundation upon which to guide their students. However, the journey to that place has been a long one.

During the third century B.C., two enterprising Alexandrian physicians conducted the first recorded public dissections on human cadavers.[1] The research, led by Herophilus and Erasistratus, successfully rendered careful structural accounts of the brain, liver, pancreas, and other organs. However, moral objections to human dissection restricted most subsequent investigations to animals.[2] The ban against cutting open a human body continued for the most part throughout the western world until the fifteenth century. As a result, many erroneous ideas proliferated regarding the human body. Modes of treatment prescribed by physicians primarily followed the ancient—and dangerous—doctrine of humoral imbalance espoused during the fifth century B.C. by Hippocrates, "the Greek father of medicine." According to the theory, the source of illness was caused by the de-synchronization of the four bodily humors: blood, phlegm, choler or yellow bile, and black bile. In order to restore the body's overall balance, physicians regularly prescribed heroic measures including bloodletting, blistering, and the ingestion of toxic substances, often to the great misfortune of the patient.[3] However, many cases necessitated surgery, including the removal of abscesses, tumors, or diseased limbs. Professional taboos regarding the cutting open of another human meant that physicians assigned such messy and repugnant work to barber-surgeons, who conducted surgery as a sideline to cutting hair and shaving beards. The familiar red-and-white poles outside barbershops originally signified the bandaged and bloodied stick given to patients to grip during minor surgical procedures.[4] In the manner of other tradesmen, barber-surgeons learned their craft through an apprenticeship rather than academic instruction. For this reason, surgeons traditionally assumed the title of "Mister" rather than "Doctor." Only physicians were entitled to call themselves "doctor of medicine."[5]

A revolutionary turning point occurred under the influence of the distinguished and controversial Scottish surgeon and anatomist, John Hunter (1728–1793). As chief surgeon of St. George's Hospital in London, Hunter determined to move the surgical profession out of the barber's chair and into the clinical laboratory by abandoning the hands-off traditions of the medical establishment in favor of in-depth anatomical exploration. With knife and forceps, Hunter spent many winters in his laboratory bent over human cadavers, discovering the intricacies of the human body while negating conventional medical theories and myths.[6] His efforts made surgery a science, grounding the future of the profession upon the doctrines of observation, experimentation, and the application of physical evidence.

Hunter's revolutionary expertise attracted an important following. Beginning with his early years in the profession, Hunter gave lectures on applied anatomy and surgery from his residence in the Covent Garden and later Leicester Square sections of London. Aspiring medical students throughout the British Isles and across the Atlantic flocked to Hunter's side, eager to study under one of the best skilled surgeons of the era. Noteworthy pupils include Edward Jenner, who would later develop the smallpox vaccine, and Joseph Lister, medical pioneer in the use of antiseptics. Many of the leading medical lights of colonial America also owed their early training to Hunter's teaching. Among them were John Morgan (1735–1789), William Shippen (1736–1808), both founders of the University of Pennsylvania Medical School, and Philip Syng Physick (1768–1837), considered the "Father of American Surgery." Through each of these men, Hunter's influence passed to succeeding generations of medical students and surgeons. However, perhaps more than anyone else, it was Physick who imported the ideals of John Hunter to the United States. As professor of surgery at the University of Pennsylvania, Physick became famous for instructing his students to "observe, deduce, and record" in true Hunterian fashion.[7]

Since Hunter's time, the surgery profession has progressed radically in terms of effectiveness and prestige. Beginning in the mid-nineteenth century, fresh discoveries and experiences spurred new approaches to the human condition. Studies obtained in the Victorian anatomy laboratory brought about the first human blood transfusion, the first successful appendectomy, and the first successful heart surgery. Military assignment to the battlefield provided an excellent training ground for would-be surgeons, exposing them to bodily conditions rarely encountered in peacetime. The development of anesthesia substantially reduced the violence of the operating room, giving surgeons the time and concentration to perform more complex, precise maneuvers than they dared contemplate before. The acceptance of aseptic and antiseptic practices significantly lowered the patient mortality rate. Each discovery, opportunity, and invention has aided the continual quest for better treatment and prevention of disease. As surgery became a dynamic contributor to medical advancement, the professional caliber of surgeons rose as well. By 1920, the possession of a university medical degree, thus earning the title of "Doctor," became essential to surgical practice.[8]

While it is highly reflective of the general history of the field, the story of surgery in Texas is also unique. Since the 1500s when shipwrecked conquistador Cabeza de Vaca removed an arrowhead from the chest of an Indian, Texas surgeons have made profound contributions to the evolution of medicine as well as the political health of their state. Many rendered battlefield service during the Texas Revolution. Seven surgeons were present at the Alamo, while others attended soldiers at Goliad and San Jacinto.[9] The expertise of Dr. Alexander Ewing is often credited for saving the life of Gen. Sam Houston shortly after he led the Texans to victory at the battle of San Jacinto. Having studied medicine at the College of Surgeons in Edinburg, Ewing was serving as surgeon general of the Texas Army when he detected the seriousness of the leg wound Houston sustained during the battle. At Ewing's insistence, Houston was sent to New Orleans for further treatment. Two years later, Dr. Ewing helped found the Medical and Surgical Society in Houston, the first effort towards organized medicine in Texas.[10] Physicians played important roles in frontier communities, and several attained high office. Dr. Branch T. Archer, a graduate of the University of Pennsylvania, served as Secretary of War in the Republic of Texas. Elected the fourth president of the Republic, Dr. Anson Jones presided over the formal annexation of Texas to the United States.[11]

Although medicine remained an archaic enterprise throughout much of the nineteenth century, many progressive-minded Texas citizens supported the creation of a medical school in their state. The prime mover behind the initial effort was Dr. Greensville Dowell. A graduate of Jefferson Medical College in Philadelphia, Dowell arrived in Galveston as a Confederate Army surgeon during the Civil War. Rather than return east at war's end, Dowell remained in Galveston, opened a practice, and launched a mission to set the Texas medical community apart from others in the Southwest. Dowell wrote extensively and published the *Galveston Medical Journal,* the first medical periodical in the state.[12] In late 1865, the Galveston Medical College opened its doors. Through a series of classroom lectures and demonstrations, local physician "professors" sought to instill high standards of medical professionalism. Students took required courses in anatomy, chemistry, obstetrics, therapeutics, and physiology, among other subjects.[13] Although the school eventually succumbed to red ink, it paved the way for a permanent endeavor led by the colorful Dr. Ashbel Smith. Having obtained three degrees from Yale, including an MD, before the age of twenty, Smith traveled to Texas in 1837, became the roommate of Gen. Sam Houston, and succeeded

Alexander Ewing as Surgeon General of the Texas Republic. During the deadly yellow fever epidemic that swept Galveston in 1839, Smith tended the sick and wrote a treatise on the disease. He traveled to Europe as the chargé affaires of Texas to England and France, a position he held from 1842 to 1844. During the Civil War, Smith led a regiment of soldiers and was captured at the fall of Vicksburg. Throughout his long career, Smith labored tirelessly to ultimately accomplish the goal of his life: the establishment of The University of Texas and an accompanying medical school, The University of Texas Medical Department. Opened in October 1891, the institution known today as The University of Texas Medical Branch (UTMB) at Galveston was housed within a beautifully ornate red brick building, designed by architect Nicholas C. Clayton. Fondly nicknamed, "Old Red," the building was later officially named in Smith's honor.[14]

Determined to set high standards for the new medical department, The University of Texas Board of Regents carefully selected the first faculty. Resisting convention, the regents chose an eclectic mix of energetic, idealistic, and talented physicians to fill the positions. Two of those selected, William Keiller and James Thompson of Great Britain, brought to Texas the best of Old World medical traditions in anatomy and surgery. Before their acceptance of the positions in Galveston, both professors had earned distinction as fellows at the Royal College of Surgeons. A graduate of Edinburgh University, the Scottish William Keiller pioneered important aspects of modern anatomy. In 1898, he introduced the formalin method of preserving cadavers and devised a system of embalming that continued to be implemented in medical school laboratories for almost a century. Keiller was also an original advocate of local anesthesia. To prove his point, Keiller insisted on having his appendix removed under local anesthesia and showed up to conduct his classes a few days later.

James Thompson, a graduate of the Manchester School of Medicine, was the first physician in Texas to limit his practice exclusively to surgery. Following the Hunterian model, Thompson used an anatomical foundation to build his approach to surgery, conceiving many of his groundbreaking operations in the anatomy laboratory. His pioneering efforts concerning congenital anomalies, particularly cysts of the neck and cleft lip and palate, have become classics in plastic surgery.[15]

For fifty years, UTMB remained the sole medical school within The University of Texas system. Only one other institution, the private Baylor College of Medicine (1903), trained physicians in Texas. By mid-century socioeconomic growth throughout the state necessitated a change. Following World War II, Texas experienced an explosion in population, urbanization, and industrialization. The oil industry and manufacturing opportunities drew millions of individuals to urban areas throughout the Lone Star State. By 1960 almost 65 percent of the Texas citizenry lived in cities. As a consequence, the two existing medical schools struggled to produce enough graduates to meet the expanding demographic. Confronting a statewide doctor shortage, The University of Texas established two new schools. In 1959, the Texas legislature authorized The University of Texas Medical School at San Antonio, which opened for classes in 1966. The dynamic growth of the Texas Medical Center encouraged the establishment of The University of Texas Medical School at Houston in 1969.[16] One of the most successful components of the Medical School is the Department of Surgery. The following chapters chronicle the historical evolution of this department and its lasting contributions to health care, education, and practice.

What can be concluded from the development of surgery as a science and as a profession? The field of surgery has been largely shaped by two trajectories. The first involved continual scientific experimentation and knowledge creation. This has resulted in a formalized scientific discipline. The second trajectory concerned surgeons as social actors and activists addressing the human condition on the battlefield and in the operating room. The confluence of these two trajectories has resulted in a highly respected and esteemed profession that has done much to alleviate human suffering and pain. The story of the Department of Surgery at The University of Texas Medical School at Houston mirrors these two trajectories. And it all began on a June day in 1969, when Gov. Preston Smith signed the bill formally creating the new medical school in Houston.

CHAPTER I

Starting from Scratch

A New Medical School for Houston

When Houston's newspapers announced on May 25, 1969, that the state legislature had approved a University of Texas Medical School for the city, the news set off a chain of events that reverberates to this day. State and local leaders fully expected that the new medical school, to be built in the Texas Medical Center (TMC), would become a successful institution having a broad impact on the region's economy as well as in scientific research, education, and patient care. Today, The University of Texas Medical School at Houston, is one component of a larger entity known as The University of Texas Health Science Center, Houston or UTHealth, located in the heart of the Texas Medical Center, a sprawling network of educational, research, and patient care institutions comprising the largest medical complex in the world. The University of Texas had a key role in creating the Medical Center, with its M. D. Anderson Hospital for Cancer Research and its Dental Branch comprising two of the original, founding institutions, but the medical school was not part of that initial configuration. When Gov. Preston Smith signed legislation creating The University of Texas Medical School at Houston (House Bill 80) on June 13, 1969, the Texas Medical Center already had a medical school in the Baylor University College of Medicine, which had relocated to Houston in 1943 to become one of the founding entities. And just fifty miles down the interstate, the university had its flagship medical school, The University of Texas Medical Branch at Galveston (UTMB). Why then put another medical school in the area, to be located just a short walk across the TMC campus from Baylor? And how does a university go about the enormous task of actually creating a medical school, assembling a faculty, recruiting students, and constructing the appropriate physical plant to house the institution, all from scratch?[1]

Many Houstonians had long desired a University of Texas medical school to be located in the city. In 1923, Will and Mike Hogg had bought a tract of land adjacent to Hermann Park and Rice University, with the hope of enticing the university's medical school in Galveston to relocate inland. When it became clear that this idea was doomed to fail, the brothers sold the land to the city at cost. Years later, the M. D. Anderson Foundation purchased the tract and on February 28, 1946, formally presented the deed to the Texas Medical Center, the original 134 acres to make up the initial site. During the next twenty years, the Texas Medical Center grew in acreage, number of member institutions, and in reputation. By the mid-1960s, Texas' population had grown to the extent that there was a need for more medical doctors and a consequent need for new medical schools in which to train them. In 1965, the state's Higher Education Coordinating Board requested that The University of Texas System conduct a study to determine the state's medical needs, projecting forward to 1990. The study group, known as the Central Committee of the UT Medical Systems Survey, was comprised of representatives from the university's health-related units—UT Medical Branch in Galveston, Southwestern Medical School in Dallas, and UT San Antonio—and was chaired by Dr. Charles "Mickey" LeMaistre, professor of internal medicine at UT Southwestern. Years later he recalled that the committee was charged to look at "manpower [and] research activities, and identify how all the medical units of The University of Texas could be enhanced, and have all of the existing health components participate to see what more they could do before we created anything new."[2]

These were exciting times in medicine and in health care in the United States. During the 1940s, medical schools began taking a major role in research, in addition to their traditional role of training new physicians. Breakthroughs in medicine and in the role of medical schools during World War II began a massive change in the scope of medical research in the US. The Office of Scientific Research and Development provided grants and contracts with the federal government during the war years, funding that continued and grew during the 1950s and 1960s. Results of research during the war contributed to public enthusiasm for continued funding and raised expectations and hopes for further advances against chronic diseases. Postwar affluence, the growth of industry, and advances in other sciences, along with the Soviet Union's challenge in space exploration (*Sputnik*, 1957), all contributed to the notion that scientific research was key to the nation's continued prosperity and world leadership. A mechanism for funding medical research was already in place. In 1930, the National Institute for Health was organized, followed in 1937 by the creation of the National Cancer Institute. In 1948, Congress enacted legislation that authorized the surgeon general to create new institutes to focus on major diseases. The addition of the National Heart Institute and the National Institute for Dental Research in 1948 led to the name change to National Institutes of Health (NIH). Headquartered in Bethesda, Maryland, the NIH was instructed to conduct research and to support research at medical schools, teaching hospitals, universities, and other places through a system of grants and contracts. Historian Kenneth W. Ludmerer, in his seminal work on the history of American medical education during the twentieth century, observed that, "Enabled by federal support, the 1950s and 1960s became a golden era of American medical research." A report published in 1959 by the Surgeon General's Consultant Group on Medical Education had instigated even more public pressure to open new medical schools. The report, "Physicians for a Growing America: Report of the Surgeon General's Consultant Group on Medical Education," generally known as the "Bane Report" after Frank Bane, the chairman of the consulting group, projected that by 1975, the country would have a shortfall of some 40,000 physicians. One result of this clarion call to train more doctors was the Health Professions Educational Assistance Act of 1964. The bill provided federal matching funds for new medical schools and funds for expansion of existing schools if they increased the number of new students in their programs. There was such a sense of urgency to increase the number of new physicians that the bill was revised in 1965, 1968, and 1971 to provide more funds and incentives to increase enrollments. Ludmerer noted that support for medical research also came from state governments, foundations, private donors, and corporations, yet figures from 1968 show that "the federal government accounted for 58 percent of the income of medical schools." As some have observed, because of this support for medical research, the years 1950–1970 were a period of great progress in the fight against a variety of diseases, with more discoveries through research than in all previous human history. All of these factors, then, contributed to the desire to establish new medical schools in Texas.[3]

While the Central Committee study was underway, Houstonians, including some of Hermann Hospital's doctors and administrators, also expressed their aspiration to have a new University of Texas medical school located in the Texas Medical Center. When the Baylor University College of Medicine first relocated to Houston in 1943, the school initially held classes in a converted Sears and Roebuck warehouse and utilized Hermann Hospital facilities for its students to gain clinical experience. The Hermann Hospital Estate (HHE), which ran the hospital, rejected a formal affiliation agreement, fearing that the medical school might want to exercise control over staff membership and exclude the hospital's veterans who would be returning from duty during World War II. Consequently, the medical school assisted with house staff training and treating patients at the hospital, but there was no formal teaching hospital affiliation. As the war ended, the Texas Medical Center formally took possession of the 134 acres purchased by the M. D. Anderson Foundation, as well as some additional acreage immediately adjacent to Hermann Hospital. The Medical Center gave Baylor's medical school a tract of land on which to construct its new building, which opened in 1947, while Hermann Hospital began construction of a 400-bed addition and a new medical office building across the street. Both of the new Hermann facilities opened in 1949. Two years later, the Methodist Hospital opened in the Texas Medical Center and reached an affiliation agreement with Baylor. Thus, Baylor no longer needed Hermann Hospital, and the school withdrew from its previous relationship. This resulted in a "steep decline" in applications for the hospital's house staff, and by many accounts, also marked the beginning of a slow decline in service and reputation. Dr. L. Rodney Rodgers, who became Chairman of the Department of Medicine in 1965, later wrote that he saw the need for Hermann Hospital to have a medical school affiliation and, as a graduate of UTMB, began to look toward The University of Texas.[4]

The Baylor-Methodist affiliation quickly developed training programs that exceeded what was available at Hermann Hospital, which left

Hermann struggling to keep up. By the mid-1960s, house staff morale declined along with conditions at the hospital. Rodgers gained support from the chiefs of services in the hospital for the idea of establishing a University of Texas Medical School in Houston to affiliate with Hermann. The Hermann Hospital Estate Trustees, the board that ran the hospital, previously had worked with the UT System in 1962 to develop an affiliation with the Graduate School of Biomedical Sciences, already located in the Texas Medical Center. Early in 1966, the hospital's medical staff raised with the HHE trustees the issue of bringing a University of Texas medical school to Houston to affiliate with the hospital. There were strong connections to UT among the estate's board of trustees, including regents Jack Josey, who also served as vice chairman of the UT Board of Regents, Walter Sterling, and UT alumnus John Holmes. The HHE trustees were very interested in an affiliation with UT and even offered 100 acres of Hermann Estate land to the university as a site for its medical school. In December, Rodney Rodgers discussed the idea of a new medical school with LeMaistre, who told him that the UT Board of Regents anticipated that the legislature would give its approval during the next biennial session, which would meet in January 1967.[5]

Later in 1966, LeMaistre's committee, the Central Committee of the UT Medical Systems Survey, presented its final, 200-page report, *The University of Texas Medical Systems Survey of the Current Status of Effectiveness and Projections.* The report offered several recommendations to improve management of UT's health-related institutions and also to create a new medical school at a site that would have the most resources, including a teaching hospital, clinicians, and teaching faculty. The state was not interested in creating new teaching hospitals, thus the requirement for a hospital that already was in place. LeMaistre stated, "they have required all the medical schools, subsequently, to have affiliation agreements with a private or not-for-profit teaching hospital and that those facilities be provided to the state at no cost. Such was the requirement here for the new UT Medical School at Houston."[6]

The bill to create a new University of Texas medical school failed to pass during the 1967 legislative session, but in 1969, with promises to support a medical school at Texas Tech University in Lubbock, Governor Smith's hometown, and to provide assistance for Baylor's Medical College in Houston, the issue finally passed. The University of Texas System pledged that it would not recruit the Baylor Medical School faculty while they were still full-time at Baylor and also to secure state funds to put Baylor's medical students on the same tuition schedule as UT. The idea was that prospective students could choose to attend Baylor without incurring any major additional cost. The Board of Regents appointed three trustees: Jack Josey, from Houston; chairman of the board Frank Erwin, from Austin; and Dan Williams from Dallas, to coordinate efforts with UT administrators and representatives from the Hermann Estate, Hermann Hospital, and the Texas Medical Center to bring the new medical school to Houston. LeMaistre later stated, "Hermann Hospital stepping forward and offering to be the primary teaching hospital was the key, but I also recall there were other affiliated hospitals that pledged help at that time, and they are equally important. More than twice the number of beds that were needed for a new medical school was offered in advance of the creation of the school." On June 13, 1969, at a ceremony in the auditorium of the Jesse Jones Library Building of the Houston Academy of Medicine, Gov. Preston Smith signed legislation creating The University of Texas Medical School at Houston—the Brooks-Bass Medical Training Act—authorizing and directing the Regents of The University of Texas to establish and maintain the school. Guests included the UT Board of Regents, the Hermann Hospital Estate Board of Trustees, and other officials. The legislation went into effect September 1, 1969, and included House Bill 80, which authorized the new medical school, and a bill appropriating $10 million for startup in 1969–1971.[7]

Now that the state officially had established a new University of Texas Medical School, administrators and the Board of Regents began the laborious process of actually hiring faculty, recruiting students, and constructing facilities. One of the first tasks was to find the right person to serve as the founding dean. Among the early candidates was Cheves McCord Smythe, MD. Smythe came from an old, established family in Charleston, South Carolina. He was educated at Yale, served in the US Navy during World War II, and graduated from Harvard Medical School in 1947. He trained in internal medicine at the Boston City Hospital and at Bellevue and Presbyterian Hospitals in New York. He also served in the Navy during the Korean War and retired from the US Naval Reserve in

1966 with the rank of commander. Smythe had been dean of the Medical College of South Carolina and in 1969, held a faculty appointment at Northwestern University School of Medicine and was Director of the Department of Academic Affairs at the American Association of Medical Colleges (AAMC). The American Medical Association (AMA) and the AAMC were working together through a committee on medical education, part of an accreditation process for the rapidly increasing number of new medical schools in the country at that time. Smythe scheduled site visits for the committee and personally visited many of the medical schools. Because of this, he had gained firsthand knowledge of many medical schools and the latest best practices in medical education. He edited the reports from those visits in preparation for presentation to the AAMC liaison committee at the annual meetings. In the course of his work with AAMC, Smythe had become acquainted with the deans of The University of Texas' existing medical schools. At a meeting of the AAMC at Houston's Shamrock Hotel in 1968, some of these UT representatives who comprised a semi-formal search committee, invited Smythe to meet with them. They wanted to discuss whether he would be interested in being considered for appointment as the university's vice chancellor of health affairs. "We talked for half a day," he recalled years later. "I said that the skills that the job called for were not mine, were not what I was interested in." Smythe had heard rumors about a new medical school in Houston, and having a role in that was of more interest to him. "I was tired of looking at other people doing things," he stated. "I wanted to do something myself."[8]

During the fall of 1969, Smythe interviewed for the deanship of the new medical school. Rodney Rodgers, who was on the search committee, later stated: "I was greatly impressed by Cheves McCord Smythe's intellectual brilliance, articulateness, enthusiasm, and aggressive pursuit of excellence." Smythe recalled that there was some debate over whether he was the right person for the appointment. "There were some people who thought I was competent and some people who thought I was dangerous," said Smythe. "And, of course, both [were] right." The Board of Regents approved the search committee's recommendation to hire Smythe. He officially became dean, at first part-time, on January 1, 1970, and on a full-time basis in April. He resigned from AAMC and, with his wife Polly, began the search for a home. The family moved to Houston in June, and Dean Cheves M. Smythe was already busy building a new medical school, from the ground up.[9]

Smythe later said that as soon as he began to take on his new responsibilities, he felt tremendous pressure in almost every administrative aspect of building the new medical school. One source of this pressure was Board of Regents chairman, Frank Erwin, who believed that the political climate in Austin was very supportive of the new medical school, and therefore it was important to move quickly in getting the new facility up and running. "Hurry, hurry, hurry," is how Smythe remembered those early days. "When the legislature is favorable, you had better move. And therefore, [Frank] was, 'get on with it, expand the class, get started, don't waste time.' He also knew that climate would not last forever, so he was putting on a great deal of pressure to get it done now because this is when the money is going to flow." One of the early questions with which he dealt was whether, organizationally, the new medical school would be autonomous or fall under administrative control of the university's M. D. Anderson Cancer Center. "That argument fell on both sides of the question," said Smythe. "My decision was that although it would hurt initially, in the long haul, it would be better for the medical school to be autonomous." Smythe's prior experience as dean in South Carolina and his years at AAMC had given him a frame of reference for how good medical schools should be composed, both functionally and for accreditation purposes. He knew how to build programs and what it would take for The University of Texas Medical School–Houston to match up with other nationally known schools. Although he did not mind too much the pressure to move quickly, in retrospect, he later stated that, "I really believe that the institution could have avoided some of its [later] trials had it been given a little bit more time initially, had the build-up of the student body been a little bit less rapid." [10]

Smythe quickly hired a small administrative staff including Sondra Ives, Faye Viola, and Carol Sherman, and in a rented office in the medical center's library building, he set to work creating the new school. Within a few short months they had recruited the first freshman class. "I arrived and the first thing I did was to recruit nineteen students right away," said Smythe. "I did not have a weekend." Because there were no facili-

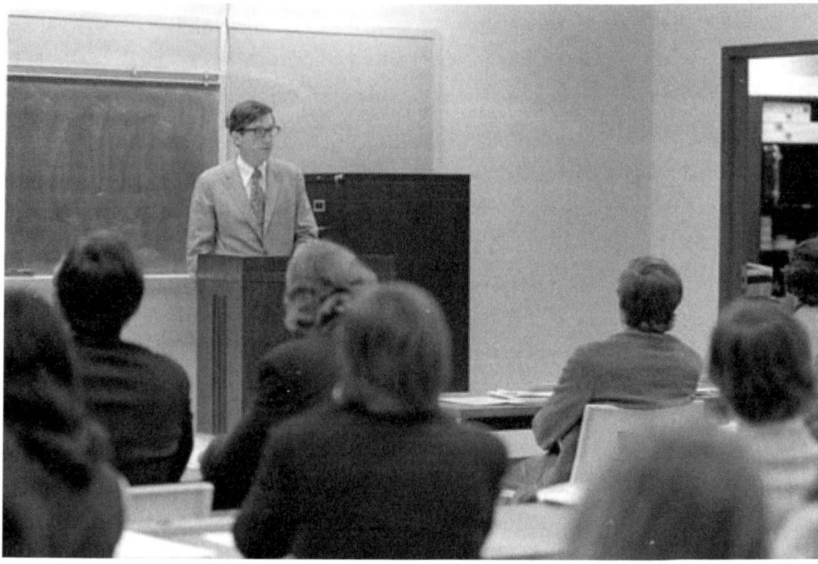

Cheves M. Smythe, MD, founding Dean, The University of Texas Medical School at Houston, presenting a lecture, 1975.

ties in Houston, students would begin their medical school careers with their first two years of study taking place at the UT medical schools in Galveston, Dallas, or San Antonio, and later, in such space as could be found in the Texas Medical Center. During this time, Smythe brought in John Bartlett as associate dean to help him manage facilities. He then began recruiting faculty and eventually convinced Robert L. Tuttle, MD, to leave his position at Bowman Gray School of Medicine at Wake Forest University and join him as associate dean at UT-Houston. Tuttle was highly regarded as a teacher and administrator and had known Smythe for many years. He joined UT-Houston in January 1971, and immediately set about establishing a curriculum and recruiting the second class of students.[11]

Smythe anticipated that his next task would be proceeding in some orderly fashion to recruit faculty and build an educational program. But soon an unexpected series of crises quickly became a major source of distraction. Smythe found himself confronted with issues related to the physical conditions in several departments at Hermann Hospital including anesthesiology, radiology, and pathology. Hermann Hospital had once been the premier hospital in Houston but by the late 1960s had fallen on hard times. There were complaints that anesthesia equipment and x-ray machines were in poor condition and that the hospital's laboratories were lacking too. Medical technology was advancing, but Hermann Hospital had not kept up. Hospital administrators' budget priorities left little for new equipment that would make the hospital attractive to younger staff, leaving the venerable old institution at a competitive disadvantage in terms of recruiting. As a consequence, younger doctors questioned why they should go to an obsolete hospital. Instead, they began choosing other hospitals, with the result that Hermann was not filling its internships. Therefore, hospital administrators welcomed the medical school, believing that it would reinvigorate Hermann.[12]

In the midst of working with the failing departments at the hospital, during June 1970, an ad hoc committee chaired by Dr. L. Rodney Rodgers discovered that the original 1968 affiliation agreement between The University of Texas and Hermann Hospital had been altered without the knowledge of the hospital's physicians. The structure of the governing boards had been changed to the extent that the hospital staff no longer had a majority on the new Executive Committee, giving control to the medical school. Many of the hospital's medical staff blamed Cheves Smythe for the changes, but as he unequivocally stated: "The affiliation agreement between The University of Texas Medical School at Houston and the Hermann Hospital was signed, sealed, and delivered one year before there was a medical school … so I had nothing to do with that." The disagreement over the affiliation agreement had ongoing repercussions. First, in 1972, several doctors on the staff at Hermann Hospital began to formulate plans to build their own medical facility (Park Plaza Hospital). Smythe did his best to mollify the feelings of the Hermann doctors, with varying degrees of success. He later recalled that he maintained personal friendships with many of them, noting, "I went to lunch with them. Our wives knew each other. I hunted and fished with many of them. We were close friends, and many of us still are close friends." The affiliation issue reared up again in 1987, when Edward Randall III, chairman of the board of the Hermann Estate, insisted on a new affiliation agreement with The University of Texas. Many of the medical school's department chairs revolted, and five eventually were fired from their positions. Years later, Richard S. Ruiz, MD, Chairman of the Department of Ophthalmology and Visual Sciences, observed: "You can imagine the immensity of trying to bring a medical school into being and to marry it to a hospital that really never had been an academic institution. I don't know many people that could have done that except Cheves Smythe."[13]

Smythe had definite ideas about the academic and social culture of the new medical school. He advocated problem-based teaching and utilizing grand rounds with actual patients for students and residents to see firsthand what they had been studying in the classrooms and laboratories. He also strongly supported the use of technology and scientific research in the school and believed that the school should play an active role in the local community. With this notion of an advanced, modern medical school in mind, Smythe reviewed the preliminary blueprints and architectural drawings for the new school and immediately concluded that the plans were "inappropriate, old, and obsolete." He pressed Frank Erwin and the other regents to abandon the plans, on which the university already had spent a considerable sum, and re-envision the campus. To accomplish this task, university officials formed a "design team" that included Smythe, architect David Graeber and some associates from his Austin-based firm Brooks, Barr, Graeber, and White, and a few people from the university's facilities staff. Charles LeMaistre, then deputy chancellor of the UT System, appointed Dr. Philip Montgomery, associate dean of The University of Texas' Southwestern Medical School in Dallas, to lead the task force. Years later, Smythe recalled Graeber and Montgomery as being significant to the success of the task force. "We put together a planning group with me and Graeber [*sic*] and Montgomery and other floating people from the facilities office in Austin, and that was the group that came up with the ideas and drawings of the Medical School. There were a lot of ideas from a lot of people put together in one planning group that worked very effectively at the time. But in terms of the design of the Medical School building, it has done us well, and they [Graeber and Montgomery] both get credit." The task force spent the next six months revising the plans for the medical school while Smythe also prepared a National Institutes of Health (NIH) grant proposal seeking federal funds available through the Health Professions Assistance Act to help pay for the construction. It was a busy time, but by June, Smythe had completed the massive grant request and eventually secured the funds.[14]

Smythe wanted to see, among other things, greater flexibility in use of space to accommodate planned and future science labs. "The prior building had a whole series of features that were built into it," said Smythe. "I perceived that many of them were already obsolete, such as the large teaching laboratories, a book bindery, of all things, zero provision for computers anywhere, and too much office space." In the end, budget constraints left many of Smythe's ideas on the drawing table. But he recognized the importance of having areas for common functions within the building. He also was concerned that for young medical students, there was no outlet for physical activities. Although he lost the concept of a floor-to-ceiling atrium in the main building, he managed to keep the Leather Lounge, a comfortable, living room type of space on the first floor, where students could gather informally to eat, visit, study, or relax. The budget forced the inclusion of large classrooms in the building but also included a spacious room on the fifth floor for entertainment and ceremonial functions, and an athletic facility on the eighth floor. Along with these major decisions regarding funding, budgets, and building design, Smythe also dealt with many details that were mundane but, in their own way, significant, including color of the carpet, use of plastic or wire paperclips, and what color IBM Selectric typewriters to order. Construction finally began on Phase I of the medical school, the two-story, 55,000-square-foot structure that would be known as the John H. Freeman Building, in August 1971. The building opened one year later and The University of Texas Medical School at Houston had a home in the Texas Medical Center. Construction soon began on the larger, 852,000-square-foot Medical School Building, scheduled to open in 1976. Meanwhile, Associate Dean Robert Tuttle scrambled to make arrangements for the thirty-two students arriving in the fall 1971 to have classroom and laboratory space. He arranged to lease rooms in the Center South Pavilion Hospital, located on Holcombe Boulevard, across from M. D. Anderson Cancer Center. The school also rented space in the Hermann Professional Building and arranged for students to study anatomy in the nearby University of Texas Dental Branch and microbiology at Baylor. Tuttle also arranged for students to gain experience in electron microscopy, using equipment that at the time was set up in a trailer outside the M. D. Anderson Cancer Center.[15]

Historian Bryant Boutwell, who compiled a thirtieth-anniversary history of the medical school, later stated about Smythe: "Cheves had a vision of what he wanted to accomplish. He had to make things happen very quickly, because they did not have any buildings. When Bob Tuttle came, he just let Tuttle loose. These guys [Smythe and Tuttle] really made things happen." Smythe later observed the urgency of the situation, saying, "When one has students staring down his throat, no faculty, no facilities, you've got to get things done."[16]

Smythe faced many challenges in recruiting faculty for a medical school that had no buildings, no onsite facilities of its own, and only promises from university administrators. "You are scrambling to pull together faculty," he said later. "You might have money, but you've got no track record, you've got no space, you have no equipment, you have no colleagues, you have no training program." Although Smythe did not view the presence of Baylor University College of Medicine as a problem, some of his potential recruits expressed doubts about it. To meet these challenges, he developed a strategy that focused primarily on people who were just coming out of training and who were seen by their peers has having high potential. Smythe used his contacts from the AAMC and everyone he had known professionally to find promising young doctors who would be willing to come into an academic program that they would be part of building, quite literally, from the ground up. He was able to recruit some established physicians, but getting "all stars" would have required more resources than he had available. "I felt one did best by targeting what I called the emerging hot associate professor rather than going after the establishment figure," said Smythe. He noted that one of the more charming characteristics of young people is their attitude of "let's get on with it, let's solve this problem. Charge the barricades!" Smythe also had a different approach to how he wanted to organize the school. Instead of having departments, he created programs that in turn would be administered not by chairpersons but rather by program directors. He wanted to establish a medical school that moved away from what he viewed as the "franchise concept of medical school organization," where people tended to view their departments territorially, like silos. Smythe's idea for an organizational structure was to create a cohesive medical school in which people worked together. He believed that the most productive scientific and clinical unit was a relatively small one in which there is a leader or a mentor, a relatively small group of people who are associated with him or her, and then the students.[17]

Several highly qualified physicians already were on staff at Hermann Hospital or held other appointments in the various University of Texas schools already in the Texas Medical Center. In time, a few joined the medical school as faculty and program directors, including Richard S. Ruiz, MD, as Director of Ophthalmology and William S. Fields, MD. Fields, a neurologist who had been on the faculty at Baylor and had subsequently relocated to Dallas, now wished to return to Houston. Smythe also succeeded in recruiting a number of highly qualified faculty and program directors over the next few years, including: Joseph Wood, PhD, neurobiology and anatomy; Walter M. Kirkendall, MD, internal medicine; John A. DeMoss, PhD, biochemistry and molecular biology; Malcolm Skolnick, PhD, biomedical communications; Marvin Chernosky, MD, dermatology; Jack Haley, MD, family practice; Herbert DuPont, MD, infectious disease; Adolph H. Giesecke Jr., MD, anesthesiology; Berel Held, MD, obstetrics and gynecology; H. John Van Peenen, MD, pathology and laboratory medicine; R. Rodney Howell, MD, pediatrics; G. Alan Robison, PhD, pharmacology; Eugene D. Jacobson, MD, physiology; Louis A. Faillace, MD, psychiatry and behavioral sciences; Gerald Dodd, MD, radiology; and Emil Steinberger, MD, reproductive medicine and biology. To launch his surgery program, Smythe wanted to bring in a young surgeon from the University of Pennsylvania who had caught his attention: Stanley J. Dudrick, MD.[18]

Stanley J. Dudrick fit the mold for the kind of young, talented, rising star for whom Smythe was searching. A native of Nanticoke, Pennsylvania, Dudrick graduated cum laude in 1957 with a bachelor of science degree in biology from Franklin and Marshall College in Lancaster, Pennsylvania. He attended the University of Pennsylvania School of Medicine, where he graduated in 1961. He then began a rotating internship and residency training in general surgery at the Hospital of the University of Pennsylvania and served as Chief Resident in Surgery under the highly regarded Dr. Jonathan E. Rhoads. After he completed his residency in 1967, he accepted an appointment to the faculty at Penn, rising from Instructor to Professor of Surgery in just five years, and was appointed Chief of Surgery at the Veterans Administration Hospital in Philadelphia. Dudrick also was deeply involved in research in hyperalimentation, or parenteral nutrition, which loaned prominence to his name within the surgical field.

The development of parenteral nutrition—the intravenous delivery of nutrients—was a tremendous step forward in terms of surgical patient care and management. The concept had been around for centuries dating back to the discovery of the circulatory system by William Harvey in 1628, and several decades later, Sir Christopher Wren's experiments involving IV infusions of alcoholic beverages in a dog gave the idea validity. However, it would take another 350 years of basic and clinical research to successfully develop parenteral nutrition from imaginative concept to genuine practice. By the 1950s, most clinicians were very aware of the problems associated with surgery and patient malnutrition. The mortality rate of malnourished post-surgical cases was in the range of 40 to 60 percent. However, this high-risk average was not due to the surgical procedure itself, but from complications, many due to the inability of patients to eat. Without a proper means of getting nutrition to the patient, many succumbed to literal starvation. Moreover, good nutrition held implications for the ability of wounds to heal properly, the incidence of infection, and other complications.[19]

By the early 1960s, Jonathan Evans Rhoads, Chairman of the Department of Surgery at the University of Pennsylvania, began to investigate the issue. A dedicated surgeon, Rhoads hated to lose his patients to the effects of malnutrition and was determined to stop it. His research resumé was already impressive. A pioneer in the study of coagulation and the use of vitamin K, Rhoads was one of the first physicians to implement sulfa drugs in the treatment of burns and peritonitis. Rhoads's search to identify appropriate diet and ways to deliver that diet to malnourished patients required extensive experimentation. The proper level of IV (glucose) sugars needed to be determined, as well the amount of diuretics to rid the body of fluid build-up. These investigations led to one predom-

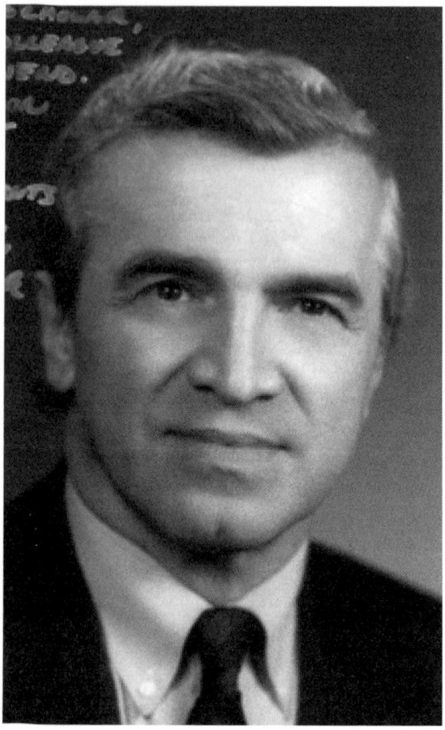

Stanley J. Dudrick, MD, founding Chairman, Department of Surgery

inant question: What was the best way to deliver the large volume of hypertonic nutritional fluid necessary for the safeguarding and healing of surgical patients? In search of answers, Rhoads's recruited his research fellow, Stanley Dudrick, to conduct the crucial experiments.[20]

Using beagle puppies as test subjects, Dudrick sought to demonstrate that proper nourishment delivered solely by intravenous infusion could have very positive results. Joseph Corriere, then a fellow researcher at the University of Pennsylvania, well remembers life in the Rhoads lab that particular year. "Stanley was in lab the year I was in lab," recalled Corriere. "As a matter of fact, I shared a cubicle with his dogs. We had a partition up, and his dogs were in one and my lab and my work was done in the other.... [H]e took a bunch of beagles, and half of them he fed normally and half they were allowed to have water . . . and then all they got was their oral nutrition through IV hyperalimentation, which meant that Stanley had to come in every day. He had been there almost twenty-four hours a day for one year or so to change this, and if a dog got in trouble, he had to fix it, and he really proved that you could do this." The beagle puppies not only survived with this method, but grew as normally as their fellow canine subjects who were fed naturally by mouth. The success of the experiment paved the way for the crucial step: testing the procedure on humans. In 1966, Dudrick and fellow researcher Douglas Wilmore treated an infant suffering from atresia of the jejunum and distal colon. The result of nourishing the child solely by vein mirrored the earlier tests on dogs. The baby recovered, gained weight, and grew normally. The studies had monumental impact.[21]

As Dr. Seymour I. Schwartz wrote in *Gifted Hands: America's Most Significant Contributions to Surgery:*

> In a landmark paper published in 1968,[22] Stanley Dudrick and associates observed six puppies that were fed entirely intravenously for 72 to 256 days and compared them to their orally fed littermates. The intravenously fed puppies outstripped their controls in weight and equaled them in development. Intravenous alimentation was then extended to human patients with success. The essence of the contribution was the threading of the catheter from the external jugular vein in the neck into the superior vena cava, which had sufficient dimensions and flow to permit the infusion of a hypertonic, high-caloric fluid without clotting the vessel. The birth of total parenteral nutrition (TPN) was critical in the expansion of surgery. This work was conducted under the direction of Jonathan E. Rhoads, professor and chair of surgery at the University of Pennsylvania and one of the giants of American Surgery.[23]

With the use of intravenous nutrition, the mortality rate of surgery patients plummeted from some 40 to 60 percent to approximately 5 percent. Witnessing the breakthrough as a young resident, Bruce MacFadyen appreciated the significance: "I thought, 'This is unbelievable that these people who came in very, very malnourished had their nutritional status replenished and survived multiple surgical procedures and stresses and strains of some of those complications.'" In other words, Dudrick proved that proper patient nutrition mattered. Whether patients faced major surgery, extensive chemotherapy, or other invasive treatment, the intravenous administration of a sound diet throughout the treatment process heightened their chances for a high quality, productive life afterward. A new era in the history of surgery had begun. [24]

Although Smythe naturally considered several candidates to lead the Department of Surgery, in his mind, Stan Dudrick absolutely epitomized his strategy of recruiting young, dynamic people for the medical school. In addition, Smythe knew Jonathan Rhoads very well and later said that Rhoads strongly supported recruiting Dudrick to Houston. Years later, Smythe recalled, "Stan had it all. He was charming. He was magic, talking to patients and their families. He had good hands. He was persistent, could stay with it." Smythe noted that Dudrick would bring with him "youth, energy, vigor, research orientation, a strategy for hyperalimentation, a plan to staff it, other young people, and recognition of the role of trauma." Smythe wanted the UT program to carve out its own niche in the Texas Medical Center, and with vascular surgery booming in the persons of Dr. Michael DeBakey and Dr. Denton Cooley, and with M. D. Anderson leading the way in oncologic surgery, Smythe saw in Dudrick not only the right man to lead the Department of Surgery, but also someone whose interest in hyperalimentation or total parenteral nutrition would be a perfect fit in the local medical community. His own surgical training had been dominated by Dr. Francis Moore in Boston, who also had an interest in studying the metabolic effects on surgery. Thus, with this frame of reference, Smythe recognized the significance of Dudrick's research. "That was what Dudrick was doing," said Smythe. "So, not only did the man fit but his interest fit the locale."[25]

During the late fall of 1971, Dudrick received a letter from Smythe indicating that a search committee had identified him as a strong candidate to lead the new Department of Surgery and inviting him to Houston for an interview. "I was extremely busy and I was certainly not looking for a job," Dudrick recalled years later. "I had the absolute best job in the Department of Surgery at the University of Pennsylvania. I had more patients than I knew what to do with at times, and it was a magnificent five years for me, the most productive five years of my life." About two weeks later, Dudrick finally arranged his trip to Houston and also went to discuss the opportunity with Rhoads. Rhoads indicated that while he hoped Dudrick would stay at Pennsylvania, he understood why he might want to go someplace new. He asked Dudrick if he would stay on at Penn until he finished his tenure as chairman, at the end of June 1972. Rhoads knew Cheves Smythe through the AAMC and had encouraged Smythe to recruit Dudrick. Thus, with Rhoads' blessing, Dudrick made arrangements to visit Houston. When he arrived in Houston he was amazed with how new, modern, and clean the city appeared, and he recalled being "a bit overwhelmed" with the size of the Texas Medical Center. The University of Texas Medical School did not yet have a building, and the staff was temporarily quartered in rented space at the edge of the medical center. They would soon move into the first floor of the Jesse Jones Library Building, close to where construction was beginning on the first structure of the UT Medical School, the John H. Freeman Building.[26]

Dudrick met with Dean Smythe, whom he found to be "very dynamic," and then with other officials from the medical school and Hermann Hospital. "I was enamored with the prospect of building a school from the bottom up," he said. On the return flight to Philadelphia, Dudrick, who was very impressed with both the city and the new medical school, later recalled, "I was really trying to process all of this information … I do not think I slept at all on the plane or at home when I got back. I just had to

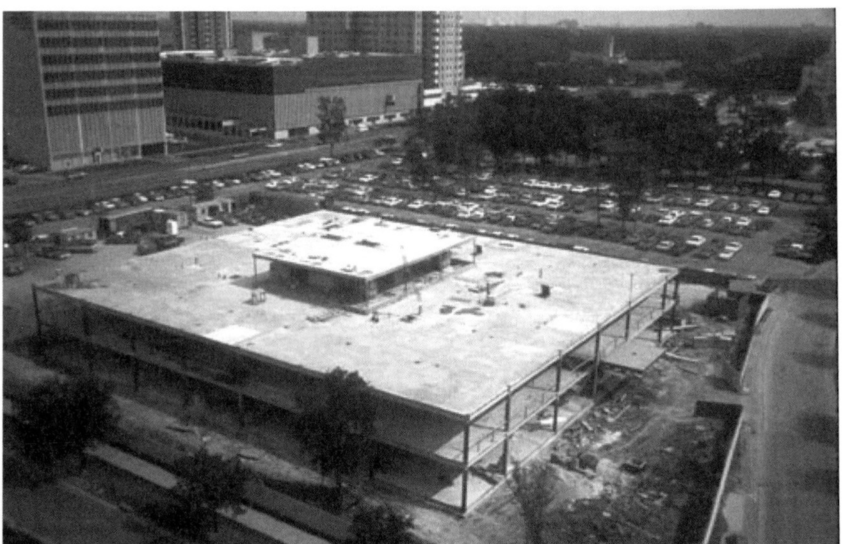

John H. Freeman Building under construction, 1972.

wait and see what was going to happen."[27]

As Dudrick returned to Philadelphia and 1971 drew to a close, Smythe could look back on two years of hard work and enjoy a moment of satisfaction. He had taken the first important steps in launching a new medical school, brought in several directors to lead the academic programs, successfully began recruiting faculty, organized the medical school, and recruited the first two classes of students. Construction finally was underway on the Freeman Building, which by the end of the following year, 1972, would be ready for occupancy as the first building on site for The University of Texas Medical School at Houston. But, students were about to begin attending classes in Houston, and Smythe needed to have all of the medical school's programs (departments) staffed and ready. More faculty needed to be hired, curriculum developed, and arrangements made for facilities, laboratory space, and equipment. Thus, there was much left to do and many questions remained, including whether Smythe had done enough to entice Stan Dudrick into uprooting his family and making the move to Houston to become the founding director of the school's surgery program. The next few months would set The University of Texas Medical School and its nascent surgery program on a path that would determine the future success of both, test the mettle of Cheves Smythe as dean, and present Stanley J. Dudrick with one of the most momentous decisions of his life.

CHAPTER 2

Building a Department

The First Recruits

By January 1972, Dr. Cheves M. Smythe, founding dean of The University of Texas Medical School at Houston, no doubt was amazed at how quickly the previous two years had passed. Smythe already had accomplished much in laying the foundation for the new institution. Many of the necessary pieces were now in place: he had hired an initial staff, recruited the first two classes of medical students, and revised the architectural plans for the medical school's nearly 900,000–square foot main building. Additionally, construction was well underway on the first of the medical school's buildings, a two-story, 55,000–square foot structure located in the heart of the Texas Medical Center, and it was on schedule to open by September. The first group of students to do all four years of their course work and training in Houston would arrive to begin the new academic term on July 1. Although Smythe had in place several program directors (department chairs), he still had several key leadership positions to fill, including some in the Department of Surgery. Meanwhile, in Philadelphia, Smythe's leading candidate to chair the surgery program, Dr. Stanley J. Dudrick, was preparing for a trip to Switzerland for a three-week visiting professorship at the University of Basel. Following his first interview at The University of Texas Medical School in Houston, he had returned to Philadelphia to reflect on all the opportunities available to him if he were offered the chairmanship of the department of surgery. Within a few days of his return from Houston, Cheves Smythe had called to follow up but made no offer, and Dudrick made no commitment. Dudrick went to Europe, where he gave his lectures and then was joined by his family to go skiing in the Alps. Here, in addition to enjoying the beautiful mountain scenery, Dudrick had time to reflect and consider his options. He realized that moving to a new environment offered a great professional opportunity and that the challenge of establishing a department of surgery in a new medical school most likely was a once-in-a-lifetime occasion. While he entertained offers from other medical schools, Dudrick was pleased when, shortly after returning from Switzerland, he was invited for a second interview in Houston.

During this return visit, Dudrick talked in detail about how he would organize the new department, his ideas about recruiting faculty, and his philosophy of teaching. He stressed that he was very much a team-oriented person. "I thought that what I would like to do in Houston is show that a group of young people could start a medical school and could express themselves and their ideas in a team fashion," said Dudrick. "My job, as I foresaw it, was to do everything I could within my ability and resources available to help all the students, residents, and faculty to achieve their God-given, maximum potential." Dudrick also stated that he wanted to build a department in which every surgeon was not only a specialist in his or her chosen area, but also had an interest in nutrition and metabolism, an area that he could continue to develop based upon his years of research in hyperalimentation at Penn. Finally, he said that he wanted to engage all of the basic scientists and the other specialties that were not surgical in collaborative nutritional and metabolic projects. His ideas clearly fit the vision that Cheves Smythe had for the medical school, and Dudrick returned to Philadelphia with a job offer in hand.[1]

Although he was inclined to accept the offer from The University of Texas, he had not formally committed to it. Smythe, perhaps sensing some uncertainty, called Dudrick, hoping to quickly arrange another meeting. But Dudrick was being inducted into the John Morgan Society at Penn and had committed to giving a paper at the ceremony that Friday in the Faculty Club. He promised to get in touch with Smythe after the weekend to set up another meeting. Following the ceremony and dinner on Friday evening, as Dudrick walked through the Faculty Club lobby to exit the building, he spied Cheves Smythe sitting in one of the leather chairs, reading a book. A surprised Dudrick realized that Smythe, who had been traveling at the time, had gone out of his way to make a stop in Philadelphia in order to recruit him to the Medical School. He invited Smythe to spend the night at his home, where the two men talked until late in the night. "We kind of bonded and I really liked him, admired him," said Dudrick. "He was just one of the smartest people I have ever known: a quick mind. At any rate, we had a marvelous evening and in the morning he went back to Houston."[2]

Since, the medical school was on a three-year program, the new term began July 1, and Smythe wanted Dudrick to be on duty to launch the new Department of Surgery when the students arrived. But Dudrick had been named a James IV Traveling Scholar, an honor awarded by the James IV Association of Surgeons. The association, founded in 1957 to create closer ties between the surgeons of the United States and England, was named after King James IV of Scotland, who had been known for his interest in science and in surgery. The association sponsored visiting fellowships for outstanding young surgeons of member countries to "promote the exchange of surgical knowledge" as well as to foster friendships among surgeons of the member countries. As a James IV Traveling Scholar, Dudrick would be presenting a series of lectures overseas and would not be available to work in Houston until mid-August. During the next few weeks, Dudrick firmed up his plans. First, he would fulfill his commitment to Dr. Rhoads by staying at Penn until June 30, the end of Rhoads's tenure as chairman, and then he would take the next six weeks to meet his obligation as a James IV Traveling Scholar.[3]

Dudrick had not told anyone at Penn that he definitely was going to Houston, because he still had a few details to work out for the position. Once he committed to joining The University of Texas Medical School, Dudrick informed Dr. Rhoads and also asked Rhoads's approval to invite Dr. Bruce MacFadyen, his resident at the VA hospital, to join him. Bruce V. MacFadyen Jr. earned a bachelor's degree in 1964 at Wheaton College in Illinois and graduated from Hahnemann Medical College and Hospital in Philadelphia in 1968. He did an internship and then residency in general surgery at the Hospital of the University of Pennsylvania. In 1971, Dudrick invited him to work on hyperalimentation with him in his lab. MacFadyen was intrigued with the research and worked with Dudrick for the next two years before making the move to Houston during the summer of 1972. "And then I came down and joined the group as a fourth-year surgical resident," said MacFadyen. "But I was on the faculty at the same time, which was kind of a unique situation. So, there were four of us that really started the Department of Surgery at that time."[4]

As Dudrick began thinking about recruiting faculty for his new department, two surgeons immediately came to mind: Drs. Edward M. "Ted" Copeland and James H. "Red" Duke. Coincidentally, Ted Copeland, who had recently returned from military service in Vietnam, already was in Houston with a fellowship in surgical oncology at the M. D. Anderson Cancer Center. Copeland was born in McDonough, Georgia, and came from a long line of physicians. Among them was his uncle, Dr. Murray M. Copeland, a surgeon and cancer specialist who was widely regarded as "one of the most influential physicians in cancer medicine."[5] Ted Copeland had studied at Duke University and then at Cornell University Medical College in New York City. Following this, he went to the University of Pennsylvania for his internship and residency. Here he met Stanley Dudrick, who was two years ahead in the residency program, and the two quickly formed a lasting friendship. After a tour of duty in Vietnam, during which he was awarded a Bronze Star for gallantry, he accepted the fellowship in cancer surgery and surgical oncology in Houston at the M. D. Anderson Cancer Center. It was during this time, in May 1972, that Stan Dudrick accepted the chairmanship at the Department of Surgery at UT-Houston. Shortly after accepting the position, he called Copeland to offer him an appointment to the faculty. But, Copeland had just recently accepted a position with a surgical group in Jackson, Mississippi. Dudrick was determined, and Copeland truly wanted to work with his old friend at the new medical school, but what to do? Dudrick persuaded the chief at the surgical group in Jackson to release Copeland from his obligation. "And July 1, 1972, I became the one and only member of the Department of Surgery at UT-Houston," said Copeland.[6]

Dudrick then focused on recruiting Duke to his new team. James H. "Red" Duke was born in Ennis, Texas, located in Ellis County, south of Dallas. As a young man, he played sports and began working at an early age on a variety of jobs, from digging ditches to welding. He began his college career at Texas A&M, where he studied engineering. Following graduation in 1950, Duke joined the army and served as an officer in the 2nd Armored Division in Germany. After completing his military ser-

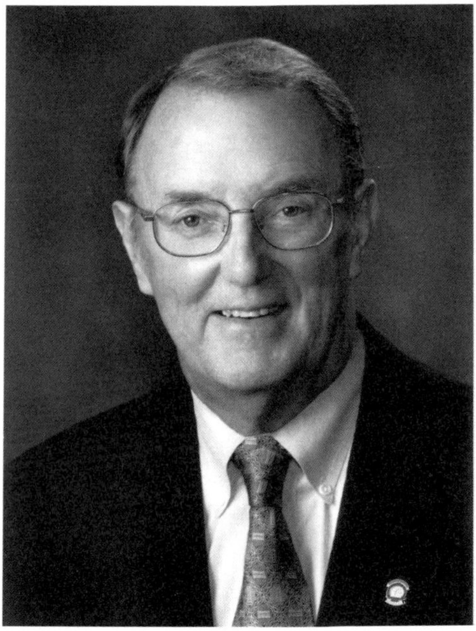

Edward M. "Ted" Copeland, MD

vice in 1952, he enrolled at Southwestern Baptist Theological Seminary in Fort Worth. Duke had been torn between the ministry and medicine since his childhood. After graduating and being ordained a minister, he realized that he still felt drawn towards medicine. Subsequently, in 1954 Duke enrolled in The University of Texas Southwestern Medical School in Dallas to determine once and for all whether to pursue a career in medicine. He completed medical school in 1960 and then did an internship and surgical residency at Parkland Memorial Hospital in Dallas. Here, on November 22, 1963, he was one of the surgeons to treat Texas governor John Connally, who had been shot during the assassination of Pres. John F. Kennedy. The following year, he became Chief Resident in General Surgery at Parkland. Duke later recalled the first time he met Stanley Dudrick, in 1965 at a Chief Residents conference in Madison, Wisconsin. "Stan and I immediately became pals," said Duke. "He was really interested in nutrition … in hyperalimentation. Well, I was really interested in that, and he and I began to cooperate." Eventually, Duke moved to New York and Columbia Presbyterian Hospital, where he received an NIH fellowship and continued his research with Dr. John M. Kinney.

Duke spent two years, 1967–69, at Columbia and frequently traveled to Philadelphia, where he was a welcome guest at Dudrick's home.[7]

Duke said that he always had an interest in being overseas and was inspired by reading about Dr. Albert Schweitzer and by Dr. Robert Shaw, who was Chief of Thoracic Surgery while he was at Parkland Hospital in Dallas. Shaw was involved with a new medical school in Afghanistan and ultimately invited Duke to join him there. From 1970–72, Duke served first as Visiting Professor of Surgery and then as Chairman, Department of Surgery at Nangarhar University, in Jalalabad. He returned to the United States in 1972 and was considering an offer to join the faculty at the University of Washington and a letter he had received from Stan Dudrick. Dudrick told Duke about his new job at The University of Texas Medical School and invited him to join the department. Although the University of Washington was very appealing, Duke agreed to come to Houston instead. "I came here because I thought that Stan and I were going to continue this really in-depth metabolic work," said Duke. "I wanted to build a better metabolic unit than they had in New York, and I enjoyed the research. That was my real intention and plan."[8]

With two top surgeons in the fold and a talented fourth-year resident, Dudrick now had his initial faculty in place and, with his family, set out on the six-week journey as a James IV Scholar. They returned briefly to Philadelphia, where he gave his last grand rounds at Penn, bade farewell, and received best wishes from his colleagues. Then he walked out the door of the hospital, climbed into his station wagon and, with family aboard and a trailer in tow, began the long drive to Houston. Eventually, two of the technicians from his laboratory and a truckload of laboratory equipment followed. Most of the equipment went into temporary storage while the Freeman Building was under construction. "We started our department on the second floor of the Jesse Jones Library building," said Dudrick. "We had one big room on the corner. You had to watch how you walked on the floor, because we had telephone cords and electrical cords crisscrossing all over, but it was marvelous. We had Ted Copeland in there and Bruce MacFadyen and the two technicians that we brought down, along with two administrative assistants—and that is how we started."[9]

Red Duke arrived a few weeks later, fascinated by the notion of hav-

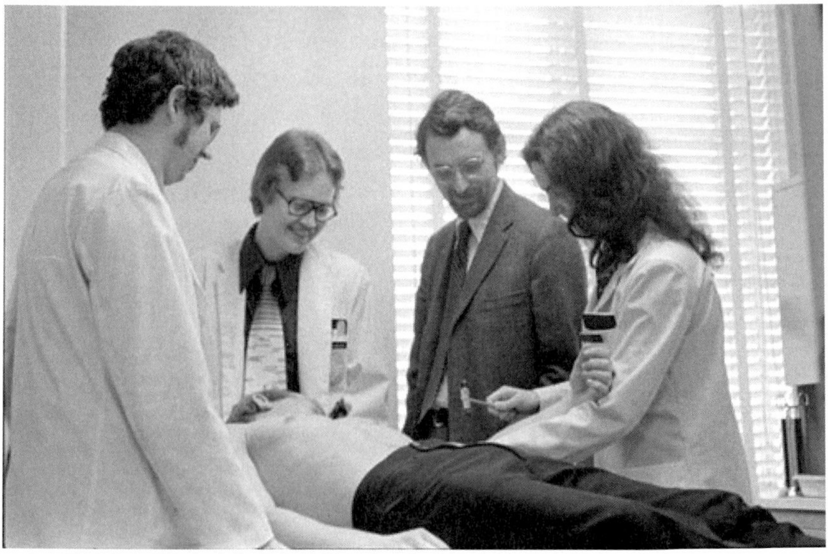

James H. "Red" Duke, MD, second from right, 1974.

ing a three-year medical school program and also that students were just now coming to Houston to study. "There were no buildings," he recalled years later. "We had some brand-new third-year medical students, and they had just now started what was called the Freeman Building. It was not even finished. What offices we had were in the library, sort of in closets."[10] Contractors had begun work on Phase I of the medical school, the John H. Freeman Building, in August 1971, and one year later, shortly after Duke arrived, the building opened. Officials and special guest George H. W. Bush, then US ambassador to the United Nations (March 1, 1971–January 18, 1973), formally dedicated the new, two-story building on October 28, 1972. The Department of Surgery was assigned to the southwest corner of the first floor, an area with space for offices, a conference room, and laboratories. After the cramped quarters in the Jesse Jones Library Building, the new suite seemed spacious and signaled the beginning of a special time for the department. "Those first years . . . I loved them," said Red Duke. "Everybody was gung-ho, starting something new, and everybody was pulling the wagon. I am talking about the [medical] school as well as the department."[11]

Ted Copeland remembered the collegiality of those early days as well, and how the fairly close quarters fostered collaboration between departments. "That was a wonderful thing, because the Department of Physiology was right there on the same floor with us and a lot of the research that all of us do is physiologically—or at least what Stanley and I do—is physiologically related." He recalled a research project with physiologist Dr. Gilbert Castro that involved studying a tape worm and using hyperalimentation or parenteral nutrition. "Gilbert became famous for that study," said Copeland. "And that was a study that was conceived just across the hall there in the Freeman Building. The point being, the beauty of being in a small building and not having many faculty is you run into each other all the time, and you could share ideas and tell jokes, and out of that may actually come something of great value."[12]

Gilbert Castro recalled that time as being like a "whirlwind" in terms of generating ideas, conducting research, and intellectual excitement. "Eventually, we did a grant together and got NIH funding to do these formal studies," said Castro. Sharing a similar interest in parenteral nutrition, surgeons and physiologists conducted numerous, cooperative studies together. Castro stated that this was, in fact, how Cheves Smythe envisioned the medical school functioning in his redesign of the main building. "His idea was to vertically separate basic sciences, put them together vertically so you could put just a straight line down this [side of the] building and on the sixth floor you would have Biochemistry; the fifth floor you would have Pharmacology; the fourth floor [surgery], you would have Physiology; the second floor was Pathology. He wanted to surround these basic scientists with clinical people so that they could interact and that they would exchange ideas." Although it did not work out to the extent planned by Smythe, on the fourth floor the surgeons and physiologists developed a rapport that led to compilation of over thirty papers during Stan Dudrick's first year as chair. "The collaboration was there and the camaraderie was there," Castro fondly recalled. "When you do these studies [with] everybody interacting together, it was unlimited what we could do. And so that is why it flourished and that is why there was that camaraderie and the fun." Castro remembered his colleagues in surgery as having amazingly positive attitudes and confidence. "Surgeons are fun to be with [and believe] they can do anything. When you come into an environment like we had at the Medical School where it was almost limitless, boundary-less, and the way Cheves had it set up, the research was boundary-less. And your interactions with people were boundary-less, and he wanted it to be that way."[13]

The typical day was busy from dawn into the night. By late afternoon, the faculty often gathered together in Dudrick's office or the conference room to discuss the events of the day. "We were not sitting around there much anyway," said Dudrick. "But every day, as much as possible, we would try to get together about 4:00 or 4:30 in the afternoon and just sit and think and share our experiences for the day and our thoughts and ideas and try to follow some sort of plan. Those were really precious times." The meetings often lasted until six or seven o'clock at night and provided the opportunity for the surgical team to discuss new ideas and form lasting bonds. Ted Copeland remembered those meetings too, recalling that Dudrick often had piles of food on the table. "It was like a fraternity meeting, quite frankly," said a bemused Copeland. "We were in the middle of Houston, Texas, surrounded by DeBakey and Cooley and all this. But there we were."[14]

The medical school's first team of surgeons faced a number of unique challenges in launching a new department at a new medical school. Their initial plan was for Dudrick, Copeland, and Duke to take turns covering the busy emergency room and trauma service at Hermann Hospital every third night, a responsibility that resulted in many sleepless nights. The doctors were concerned about the level of care being provided in the hospital's emergency room at the time. As Dudrick recalled, "We did that to get people used to the fact that there was going to be supervised treatment in the emergency department, not unsupervised house officers and nurses trying to take care of people."[15]

Soon this responsibility fell to Duke and Dudrick because of what was both a need and an opportunity that arose at M. D. Anderson. At that time, the M. D. Anderson Cancer Center had four general surgeons who did most of the general surgical procedures. During the summer, when one of the surgeons suddenly departed, the hospital was left acutely shorthanded. Copeland was offered the opportunity to fill the vacancy temporarily until they could bring in a new surgeon. Copeland recalled that Dudrick and Duke were eager for him to take on this responsibility and also to establish a departmental presence at the cancer center. The idea was that as the medical students and residents rotated through M. D. Anderson, Copeland would provide a smooth integration of services. "It meant they would have to cover the Hermann Hospital Emergency Room every other night for an indeterminate period of time," said Copeland. "That bothered me, because Hermann Hospital had just opened a big emergency room. Stanley, myself, and Red Duke were taking call every third night, and we were busy. So, for me to go to M. D. Anderson left those guys covering every other night." Years later, he reflected on what this meant for his career. "Seldom have two men and their families done so much to launch the career of a young academic surgeon," said Copeland. "For the next ten years, I had what I considered the best job in American surgery, running a medical school service at the M. D. Anderson Hospital, a category-one cancer institution."[16]

In addition to the demanding clinical schedule, the new faculty of the Department of Surgery faced other challenges. One of the first was fully integrating the surgical residents already at Hermann Hospital into The University of Texas program. The hospital had a freestanding residency program in surgery that, in the view of some, was poorly organized. As Stan Dudrick later recalled, "It was kind of a patchwork preceptorship, where it went under the name of a residency but it operated like a preceptorship. We had to try to break that up without getting everybody mad at us." Surgeons and residents at the hospital had connected with each other in a way that generally allowed them to work together with the same surgical teams. The problem with this arrangement, however, was that while the residents were working with surgeons they were comfortable with, they were not getting the kind of comprehensive training that they would receive from multiple experiences with multiple people. "And so, we had to win the residents over," said Dudrick. Another issue arose because he used the Socratic method of teaching—asking questions rather than lecturing. Some residents resisted this teaching style, while others sometimes displayed sour attitudes, in part because of negative comments from the hospital's staff and the continuing resentment of some staff toward the medical school—the town-and-gown syndrome. "It was an interesting time," said Dudrick. "These are little things that you do not anticipate until they happen."[17]

When a medical school comes to a community and affiliates with a hospital as its teaching institution, a conflict often arises between the hospital's house staff of local doctors (town) and the doctors from the medical school (gown). In most of these affiliation agreements, the medical school department chairs take over as chiefs of the service departments in the hospital. Depending on the nature of the agreement, this sometimes disrupts hospital governance, interrupts longtime clinical assignments, and in some cases displaces the local hospital staff. Some hospital physicians have little interest in taking on additional teaching responsibilities, while others expect to receive prestigious academic appointments in the new medical school. This can lead to bitter disappointment when they learn that they do not possess the appropriate academic credentials. In time these problems can be worked out, helped along by a well-planned affiliation agreement. But, in the case of Hermann Hospital and The University of Texas Medical School, this proved to be a difficult situation. Disputes arose about the affiliation agreement that stirred anger and mistrust in the hospital. "We had a disconnect that was unfortunate with this whole concept of Hermann Hospital and The University of Texas marrying each other," observed Dudrick. "It became apparent to me after a little while that this was a shotgun marriage. This was not a marriage where the component parts, meaning all the constituents, wanted to get together because they liked each other."[18]

Another aspect of the tension that simmered beneath the surface of the relationship between Hermann Hospital and The University of Texas Medical School related to the academic roles available to the hospital's physicians and surgeons. Smythe, as the medical school's dean, attempted to find a solution and provide an opportunity for the hospital's medical doctors to have a place at the school. Dudrick later recalled working with Smythe and trying to find ways to be inclusive of the hospital's surgeons while not compromising the academic standards required for the medical school's accreditation. "I do not know any of them to have any credentials to be a professor," he told Smythe. "We'd better be careful how we do this." They proposed offering a two-year blanket faculty appointment to every surgeon at Hermann Hospital as an associate in surgery at The University of Texas Medical School at Houston. This would offer those who wanted to take a teaching role in the new medical school an opportunity to demonstrate their academic proficiency and get accustomed to the academic life. Dudrick pledged that he would not crowd out the hospital staff from the department by hiring any more full-time people than necessary to carry out the didactic, scholarly, investigative curriculum requirements of the Accreditation Council for Graduate Medical Education and the Residency Review Committee in Surgery. He also stated that during the second year, he would ask these surgeons to nominate an advisory committee of five or six doctors to offer recommendations on who should be an instructor, assistant professor, associate, or full professor, and who should stay on as an associate in surgery or determine who might want to leave permanently. "I could not imagine anything more fair than that," said Dudrick. He recalled that this offer was met with mixed reactions. "Some of them were miffed that I had snubbed them," he said. Some of the hospital's surgeons believed they already had the qualifications to teach in the medical school and wondered why they had to go through this internship when they already were teaching surgical residents? Dudrick explained that with a medical school, each department had to meet specific academic standards or lose its accreditation as a medical school. Dudrick said that a small number of the physicians embraced the idea, but most did not. It was doctors from that group that created Park Plaza hospital or otherwise left Hermann for other hospitals.[19]

Sometime during 1972, six doctors began planning to build their own hospital. Dr. Henry Goodwin Glass, who had been Chief of Surgery at Hermann Hospital, later explained how he and many colleagues believed that they had lost control over their patients and the way that they practiced medicine. "We had lobbied for a medical school to be put in at Hermann Hospital," said Glass. "But when the school came in, it changed the way we practiced medicine. Our private patients were turned over to residents and interns once they were admitted to the hospital. We couldn't even write orders on the chart." Soon they had attracted twenty-two general partners and 125 limited partners in the venture. Three years later, on April 13, 1975, they opened their doctor-owned, 356-bed hospital, Park Plaza Hospital, at 1313 Hermann Drive, just down the street from the Texas Medical Center.[20]

After the initial hard feelings and a period of adjustment, however, the situation began to improve. "By that time, we were rolling along, the physical plant was getting built, and we were developing good teaching services at Hermann Hospital," said Dudrick. "We already had good people at Hermann, good surgeons and good specialists, and a good brand of medicine; they just were not professional teachers, so to speak, or investigators, but we tried hard." Dudrick stated that his goal had never been to take over Hermann Hospital or absorb it into the Medical School but to integrate the people that were there with the goals and mission and vision of the Medical School so that they could all be part of it. Even before he accepted the appointment as director of surgery, however, Cheves Smythe had warned Dudrick that he expected many of the hospital's surgeons would resent the presence of a young, Ivy League doctor and might interpret his success as failure on their part. During one of his interview visits, Dudrick had met with several of the major surgeons at Hermann Hospital, went to lunch with them, and enjoyed a generally pleasant time. "I was favorably impressed with them," said Dudrick. "I thought they were fine people, nice people." To his dismay, just three weeks after he arrived in Houston permanently, he found many of these very same people to be rude and uncooperative. They accused him of doing things that they considered to be not the "real Hermann Hospital." Referring to those early days as "the old Hermann," Dudrick later opined that the present day Memorial Hermann Hospital is a much different and vastly improved place. But of those early days, he stated, "It was harsh at times."[21]

Not all of the hospital's surgeons resisted the medical school, and Dudrick recalled, "The two most outstanding faculty that helped us at Hermann Hospital were John Perry and George Boyles. They actually became the first two clinical professors of surgery. They were marvelous, and the kids loved to work with them." Bruce MacFadyen observed that although there were many changes as the hospital's residency program evolved from a private practice training program to one which was a university training program, some of the private surgeons also participated in training the residents. "I benefited from some of those guys," said MacFadyen. "Some of them were really good and I learned a lot from them."[22]

Hand in hand with the issue of the disgruntled and departing doctors was the challenge of developing a medical practice for the residents and faculty. Since Hermann was a private hospital, when the doctors left for Park Plaza or other places, they took their patients with them. The drop in patients threatened the economic viability of Hermann Hospital and its status as a teaching hospital for the UT Medical School. The school's students, interns, and residents all needed access to large numbers of patients in order to gain clinical experience, and indeed, to practice medicine. The situation was less severe for the Department of Surgery as compared with some of the medical school's other departments. As Ted Copeland recalled, "We did not have the problem with the surgeons that the [other] guys had. Surgeons always follow their referring physician, so if their referring physicians move to Park Plaza, they've got to go down there, too. But we got along relatively well." The fact that Hermann Hospital was not highly regarded for its emergency services at this time also had an impact on the patient population. Thus there was both a need and an opportunity to create something special at Hermann Hospital. Duke, Dudrick, and Copeland believed that they could improve the emergency center and through it also increase the patient population in the hospital. They viewed the emergency room (ER) as one of the entry points into the hospital and were determined to let people know that Hermann Hospital was now going to have medical staff people in the emergency department to help residents, students, and nurses with patient care. This led, then, to the initial decision for the three surgeons to be on call for the ER. In time, this would lead to the creation of an innovative aerial ambulance service and later, Hermann's designation as a Level I Trauma Center. But in those early days of the Department of Surgery, the UT surgeons spent many nights and weekends on duty at the hospital. Hermann had only recently built a new emergency room and trauma center, and Drs. Duke, Dudrick, and, for a while, Copeland, provided a level of treatment that helped add to the hospital's patient population.[23]

Despite some of the issues related to the relationship with Hermann Hospital, most of the Houston medical community was supportive of the new medical school and helpful to its surgical faculty. Phillip Adams, who began medical school at UT-Houston in 1973, later recalled that in those days, it seemed that "the Baylor people sort of ran the town as far as the medical school goes." Adams saw this to be true both in the Medical Center and surrounding communities, because many Baylor graduates remained in Houston and established their practices in the area. "UT had to fight their way up to get some respect," said Adams. "I think the Baylor people finally realized that there was plenty of business for everybody here. Over time, it became not an issue; it was mostly cooperation." In the midst of all these efforts to establish the department, the UT surgeons worked hard not only at their jobs but also to become a part of the broader medical community. "We would go to the Texas Surgical Society meeting and the American College of Surgeons Texas Chapter, and everybody was eager to meet us," said Copeland. "We participated. We tried our best to be available and integrate ourselves in the activity of Texas, and we did." He found support from physicians and other surgeons from around the state. "Denton Cooley could not have been nicer," said Copeland. "He learned our names and we often would see him at the Southern Surgical Association meeting." He also remembered the Baylor faculty with whom he interacted as being very supportive. "Ken Mattox (Baylor College of Medicine and later Chief of Surgery at Ben Taub General Hospital) could not have been friendlier," said Copeland. "To this very day, he is a good friend." Dr. Kenneth L. Mattox recalled those days: "Compete? Yes, but we saw ourselves as cousins, as really helping them to develop, not trying to destroy them." Bruce MacFadyen remembered, "There was certainly competition for patients but there were always a lot of patients."[24]

Yet, the establishment of well-trained, energetic faculty was only half of the equation. Student and resident recruitment also mattered. The first medical school class was small, comprised of nineteen students who underwent a three-month surgical rotation. Department chair Dr. Stanley J. Dudrick and his team continued recruiting new faculty to fill out the department, training new surgical interns and residents, and providing services to the Hermann Hospital emergency room. One of the surgical residents already at Hermann Hospital was Dr. Eduardo A. Souchon, who would be one of the first residents to graduate from the Department of Surgery. Souchon, a native of Venezuela, completed medical school there in 1968. By 1970, he set out to specialize in surgical oncology and embarked on a series of interviews with several medical schools in the United States. His first stop was in Houston, where he met with Dr. R. Lee Clark, director of The University of Texas M. D. Anderson Cancer Hospital and Tumor Institute. Clark asked about Souchon's medical training and learned that in Venezuela he worked for Dr. Hermogene Rivero. Clark and Rivero had interned together at the American Hospital in Paris and were old and close friends. Clark told Souchon that UT was about to open a medical school in Houston and then called the Chief of Surgery at Hermann Hospital on Souchon's behalf. "I walked over and they received me at Hermann with a contract," said Souchon. "So, I canceled all my future interviews because once you got to the Texas Medical Center, you were overwhelmed by the immensity of it. I thought, 'If I get into the surgical program here and I have M. D. Anderson here, that will be my dream come true.'" Souchon completed an Internship and General Surgery Residency in 1976 and a fellowship in surgical oncology at M. D. Anderson Hospital and Tumor Institute in 1977. He then returned to practice and teach in Venezuela, where he stayed until 2002. In 2003, he returned to Houston to join the faculty of the UT Medical School Department of Surgery.[25]

One of the first interns the department brought in was Timothy A. Dernbach, and the following year, one year after Dudrick and the new department moved into the Freeman Building, they were able to begin a formal matching program. They recruited three new interns from the University of Kentucky: James Wallace, Michael McFee, and Charles Rodman. Dudrick recalled the Kentuckians as being "very bright and affable guys. They were extremely strong," said Dudrick. John Daly, who was a graduate of Temple University School of Medicine in Philadelphia and had worked with Dudrick during the summer months at Penn, also joined the department as an intern. "They were great role models," said Dudrick. "And in a way, those were the pillars of the department."[26]

In addition to Bruce MacFadyen, several of these early recruits have become stars in the American surgical world. After a stint as Chief of the Division of Colorectal Surgery at Memorial Sloan Kettering in New York, surgical oncologist John Daly went on to chair the Weill Medical College Department of Surgery, Cornell University, and then returned to his alma mater to become dean of the Temple University School of Medicine. Regularly ranked by his peers as one of the Best Doctors in America, another former UT surgical resident, Wiley W. "Chip" Souba, became dean of the Geisel School of Medicine at Dartmouth and editor of the surgical handbook, *ACS Surgery: Principles and Practice*, deemed the "surgeon's bible" by many in the field. The successful careers of these surgeons testify to the quality education provided by UT-Houston during those early years in the 1970s. Initially, several of the new residents came from the University of Pennsylvania, including George Benson, who arrived after fulfilling an army commitment. Bruce MacFadyen remembered this and the camaraderie it generated as a positive factor in developing the new department from scratch. "It was interesting because the style of practice, the way we handled things was all very similar," said MacFadyen. "We knew each other and so it was a unique situation from that standpoint that we were able to accomplish a lot of these things." Soon the residents were completing their training and beginning their own surgical practices and academic endeavors. Eduardo Souchon recalled, "My first year, we graduated two guys, Michael Kelly and myself. The second year was Dr. Timothy Dernbach, the only senior resident."[27]

Phillip R. Adams was another product of the University of Pennsylvania who came to Houston. "I applied to the medical school and ended up coming down here in 1973," said Adams. "That is where I met Dr. Dudrick. When I was interviewing with him he had just come from

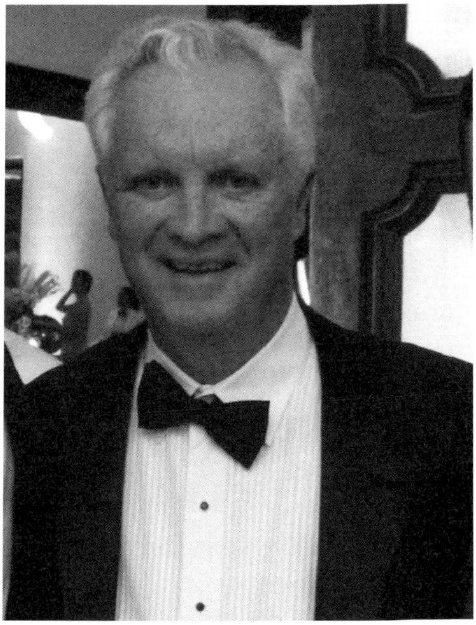

Eduardo A. Souchon, MD.

Pennsylvania and was sort of impressed by the fact that I was a Penn graduate and that I played football there." Adams recalled that at the time, the medical school was based on a three-year program of study (this changed in September 1977 when The Medical School changed to a traditional four-year program). "We went to school all year around, tri-semesters. So, for three years, we never had much of a break, maybe a week at any time. And that was nice to get done in three years instead of four." The Freeman Building was only two stories and simply was not large enough to accommodate the full medical school. This resulted in students taking anatomy in the basement of the dental school and attending some classes in other buildings around the Texas Medical Center. "The facilities were bad, but the education was good," said Adams. He recalled how Dr. Dudrick traveled frequently, giving talks about nutrition. Sometimes, he would return late in the evening, and the medical students had to be prepared to make rounds with him. "He would expect you to be there to make rounds with him at 11:00 p.m. a lot of times, even if you were on call the night before," said Adams. "I mean, there was just no excuse. Everybody had to be there."[28]

While going through medical school, Adams became interested in becoming a surgeon. He was admitted into a surgical residency at UT in 1976, and then applied for a cardiovascular and thoracic surgical residency at the Texas Heart Institute with Dr. Denton A. Cooley. "I started there in 1981 and we were doing about 4,500 open heart cases a year. So, we would do thirty-five, I remember a few days, we did fifty cases with cardiopulmonary bypass . . . I worked 120, 130 hours a week. I just operated all the time. That is how I learned how to become technically competent—because you had to be. There was just so much work to do taking care of the patients, learning how to be efficient and how to utilize your time."[29]

Adams remembered his medical school experience as being unique, mainly because of the small size of the class—about forty-eight students—and the fact that it was a three-year program at the time. "There was a small enough class that when we had the events, everybody came," said Adams. "And the faculty was very nice. They worked us hard but also entertained us and supported us." Dean Smythe was determined to create an environment in which people were "relaxed and happy at what

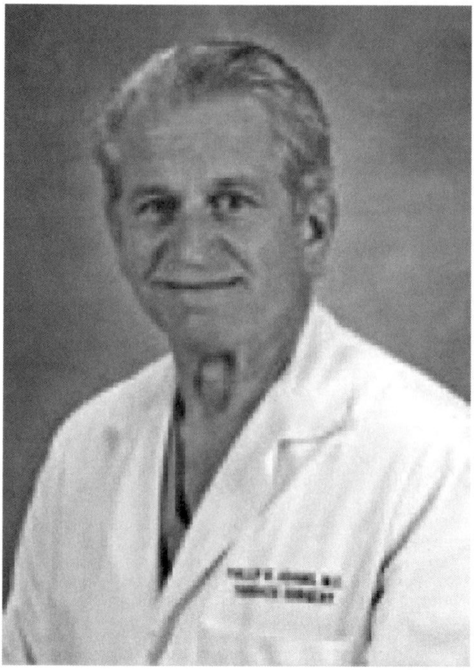

Phillip R. Adams, MD.

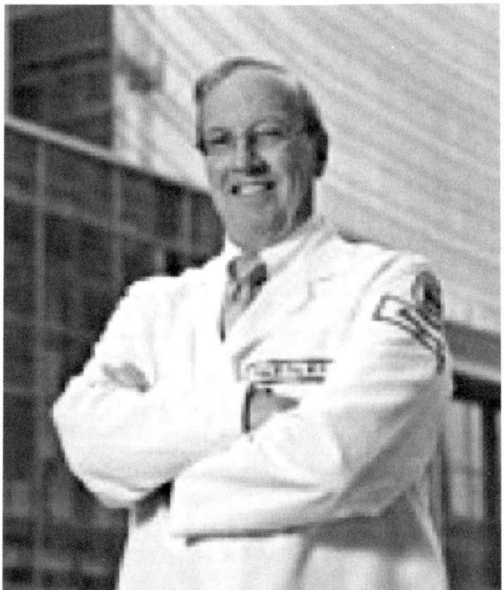

John Daly, MD.

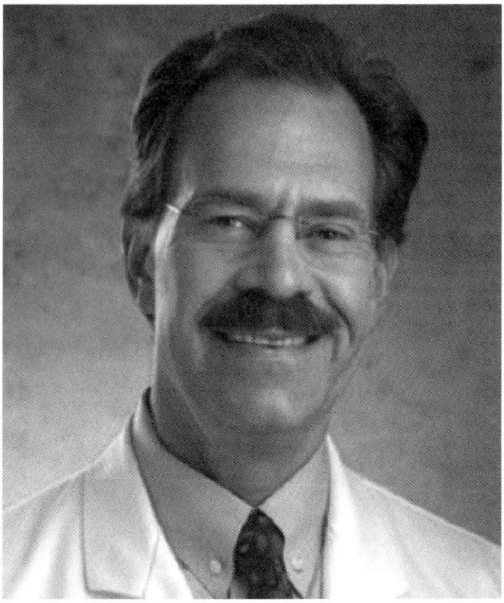

Wiley "Chip" Souba, MD.

they were doing, and in the best sense of the term, enjoy[ing] their time at work." Smythe wanted to do something to generate camaraderie and bring the faculty and students together, so in 1971, he and Polly invited the whole medical school to their home for a barbecue. "For the first two to three years, Polly and I would have a barbecue here in the backyard, and believe it not, we would ask the whole medical school. I mean, everybody—the secretaries, the clerks, the medical students." The event was very popular, but because of the growth of the school, Smythe was unable to continue the event. Several years later, however, Smythe was doing a lot of fishing and finding that he had more fish than he knew "what to do with." In the late 1980s he began a tradition that lasted almost ten years: inviting faculty and students to his home for a backyard fish fry. Historian and UTHealth faculty member, Bryant Boutwell, remembered those annual events fondly, noting: "Gil Castro and several co-hosts over the years assisted Cheves both to catch the fish and to put on the event that seemed to grow in size and popularity with each year. Cheves would take all the fish he had stockpiled in his freezer and put on one heck of a fish fry for guests who filled his backyard and house." Students appreciated the opportunity to relax, socialize with the medical school faculty, and enjoy the gracious hospitality of Cheves and Polly Smythe. As Boutwell recalled, "And, to this day, students remember ... it became quite the school event to go to the Cheves Smythe fish fry."[30]

Life as a surgical resident, then, was both lively and challenging. "It was hard work," Eduardo Souchon remembered, but "fun at the same time." A resident's day began at Hermann Hospital at 5:30 or 6:00 in the morning with early morning patient rounds. Dressings were changed, lab work and x-rays ordered, and detailed notes recorded on patient charts—all collected on paper. In those days, nothing was recorded electronically. Residents reported for duty in the OR by 7:20 to prep the operating rooms for Duke, Dudrick, and other faculty to begin their work by 7:30 sharp. Afternoons were filled with additional rounds, compiling a history and physical for all patients admitted, and other tasks. For residents, the day ended around ten o'clock at night. "My children did not know me until they were four or five years old," said Souchon. For him and others, there was no such thing as the mandated eighty-hour work week many residents experience today.[31]

The rigidity of the UT surgical resident's schedule was typical to the profession. Other resident experiences at Hermann were not. The hospital supported a clinic service, located in the original, elaborately paneled portion of the hospital. Beyond old-style double doors, clinic rooms helped poor, county patients, most of whom were unable to pay and lacked insurance. However, the UT residents handled these patients with the same regard and care as private patients. It was "a wonderful thing," noted Souchon, "As residents, we had control of all those patients. Faculty were just supervising . . . we were like the doctors . . . we would get them on the surgery schedule right behind the private cases or in between . . . That is how the interns could get to do little operations—my first appendix, my first hernia, my first hemorrhoid amputations, things like that, during those years." Residents gained additional experience assisting cardiovascular surgeries, or taking the lead in "minor" efforts including coronary bypass surgery. In this manner, early residents gained invaluable experience in a multiplicity of surgical tasks. As they progressed through the five-year residency program, residents acquired a broader range of responsibilities.[32]

Each succeeding year, then, brought more intensive training and increased opportunities for the residents to hone their skills as surgeons. Eduardo Souchon recalled, "As interns, we did not operate much, but we saw a lot. The second and third years, we did a lot more. The fourth year, we went through the rotations and specialties. The fifth year is your chief year [in which] you are supposed to organize everything … so, as you progressed, then your responsibilities got broader and broader." Phillip Adams noted that it was a brand new department with one of the youngest chairmen in the country. "Dr. Dudrick and Dr. Duke were developing their practices and they had very complicated patients," said Adams. "Dr. Dudrick, in particular, because of his studies in nutrition, always had complicated gastrointestinal problems. But, everybody was practicing and the staff and the faculty just grew, not exponentially but steadily, and the hospital along with that also increased in size."[33]

These first years of the UT-Houston department of surgery were exciting, challenging, and most definitely an eventful period for all. The department had moved from its original tight quarters in the Medical Center Library's Jesse H. Jones Building into a still cramped but slightly more spacious John H. Freeman Building. As chairman and chief of the Department of Surgery, Stanley J. Dudrick brought fresh ideas and high energy to the fledgling University of Texas Medical School. He traveled extensively, actively recruited faculty, and constructed the means to keep them. Downplaying the negatives of Houston life—the long, oppressive summer heat in particular—Dudrick promised and found the money and resources each potential faculty member required. A core faculty, including Dudrick, Edward M. Copeland, James H. Duke, and Bruce V. MacFadyen, immersed themselves in developing a surgical training program, reinvigorating emergency services at Hermann Hospital, and continuing their research endeavors. They became active in the local medical community and added a key component to the newly created University of Texas Medical School. The tireless dedication of these and other early faculty recruits laid the groundwork for a highly successful medical school program. Years later, Cheves Smythe said of Dudrick: "Stan was also a pretty good judge of talent, because you would look at the quality of the people, the initial crowd he brought with him, and what has subsequently happened to those men—he judged it right. Now, he and surgery were literally a breath of fresh air running through the hospital."

And of the original team in the department of surgery, Smythe would write: "That group of able and energetic men picked up the Hermann surgical service by the scruff of the neck, gave it a good shake, and in short order there was a respected and respectable service in place."[34]

With a foundation for their department in place, Drs. Dudrick, Duke, Copeland, and MacFadyen began to look to the future. They could now anticipate continuing their research, training new students, interns, and surgical residents, and developing new and better ways of performing surgery. The next few years would bring exciting opportunities for pioneering research in nutrition, organ transplantation, anti-rejection drugs, technology, and virtually every aspect of surgery. And a daring idea for transporting seriously injured accident victims and other critically ill patients would help put the medical school, its teaching hospital, and its Department of Surgery into the public spotlight, leading to improved emergency services and the saving of many lives, all in a very dramatic way.

CHAPTER 3

Initial Impact

The 1970s

By the mid-1970s, the faculty and staff of The University of Texas Medical School at Houston Department of Surgery were deeply engaged in establishing their presence in Hermann Hospital and in the larger Houston medical community. They had been training new students and surgical residents and also working with those who had been part of the Hermann Hospital training program. Led by their department chair, Stan Dudrick, the surgeons continued their efforts to build the department through focusing primarily on two important missions: the advancement and upgrading of acute care services (emergency surgery for individuals in need of urgent or immediate care) and a strong emphasis upon medical research. Forty years later, both missions remain the hallmarks of The University of Texas surgery program.

Modern trauma initiatives in Houston began in 1949, when Michael DeBakey brought his World War II experience developing mobile army surgical hospital (MASH) units to Baylor University College of Medicine. After linking Baylor to Jefferson Davis Hospital, DeBakey obtained a grant to establish a Trauma Research Center in Houston. DeBakey first used the term "Trauma Center" to describe the organizational structure of trauma care being implemented at the hospital. It was at Jefferson Davis that the initial concepts of emergency surgery—aggressive blood transfusion, silicone treatment of burns, aggressive fluid resuscitation, and other concepts—were inaugurated. When Ben Taub General Hospital opened in the Texas Medical Center in 1963, around-the-clock trauma teams and "shock rooms" entered the scene.[1]

During the early years, Hermann Hospital, the clinical affiliate for The University of Texas Medical School at Houston, was not considered a trauma emergency room (ER). As a young resident often working a slow shift at Hermann and looking for something to do, Eduardo Souchon remembered calling the Houston fire department EMS. "I would call the fire department because the fire department would take all the patients to Ben Taub," remembered Souchon, "So, I would call . . . and say, 'Hey, bring something here.'" Those circumstances would change in 1976 with the advent of Life Flight and later, with the subsequent designation of Hermann Hospital to a Level I Trauma Center. In consequence, a healthy competition arose with fellow surgeons at Baylor. While DeBakey and Cooley maintained very strong cardiac and vascular surgery programs at their institutions, UT surgeons gained nationwide notoriety for the trauma program implemented at Hermann. Through widespread publication, many of the concepts, standards of practice, techniques, and technology developed in Houston became the template for national and international guidelines in trauma care.[2]

By the early 1970s, then, Houston, with its rapidly growing population, also was developing an increasing need for more and better trauma care. This, in part, was on Stan Dudrick's mind when he agreed to accept the appointment as Chairman of the Department of Surgery. "The dean asked me if I would commit to paper what my vision would be and what I could possibly bring to Houston," said Dudrick. "One of those is the helicopter. That was part of my deal for coming down there: that they would support the initiation of a helicopter ambulance service and I would staff it with students and residents."[3]

Houston had begun taking steps to improve citywide emergency assistance five years earlier, in 1967, when the City Council asked the Harris County Medical Society (HCMS) to make recommendations to improve the city's ambulance services. Traditionally, area funeral homes provided transportation of sick and injured patients to local hospitals via their funeral hearses. Otherwise, injured patients sometimes were transported by private cars or by taxis that often had thick, clear plastic covers on the rear seats to keep blood and fluids from staining the material. After studying the situation and comparing Houston with other large cities, the HCMS recommended that the Houston Fire Department take over the responsibility for providing ambulance service. In 1972 the city approved this recommendation, and the Emergency Medical Service (EMS) became part of the fire department. When Red Duke arrived in Houston later that year, the EMS was still a new concept, but it captured his attention immediately. He began working with the Harris County Medical Society and helped develop an initial paramedic training program.[4]

During the ensuing months, Stan Dudrick began working to convince hospital administrators and the trustees of the Hermann Hospital Estate that the hospital should look into developing a helicopter ambulance service. Meanwhile, the UT surgeons also began working on improving the emergency room services at Hermann Hospital. Drs. Dudrick, Duke, and, for a time, Copeland, began taking call, rotating every third night and weekends. They believed that a good emergency room with a reputation for excellent patient care was one important way to increase patient flow and admissions to the hospital, which in turn would increase hospital revenue. By some estimates, the Hermann Hospital emergency services were not very highly regarded by the community, and the hospital seemed to rely more on attracting private patients who could afford to pay for their care. But as Dudrick observed: "If you want to do that, you have to be a Mayo Clinic." With construction of a new emergency room about to be completed, the timing for improved services and a helicopter ambulance fit perfectly.[5]

Now, however, with Ted Copeland doing most of his work at M. D. Anderson, the brunt of the responsibility for emergency room call fell to Duke and Dudrick. They had already begun taking steps to improve relations with the emergency responders of the fire and police departments in an effort to refurbish the Hermann emergency room's reputation. "Whenever a fireman or EMT with the fire department or a police officer would come in with a patient, we always spoke to them," said Dudrick. "Jim [Duke] or I would go. That was our policy. We would make sure we talked to the officer or whoever brought the patient in to thank them for bringing the patient and ask if there was anything we could do for them." They maintained a supply of hot coffee, donuts, and other refreshments that were available to the EMTs and police officers before they went back out on the street. As Dudrick recalled years later, "These were little things that we tried to do to make them welcome and to let them know that they were part of our team and we wanted to be part of theirs."[6]

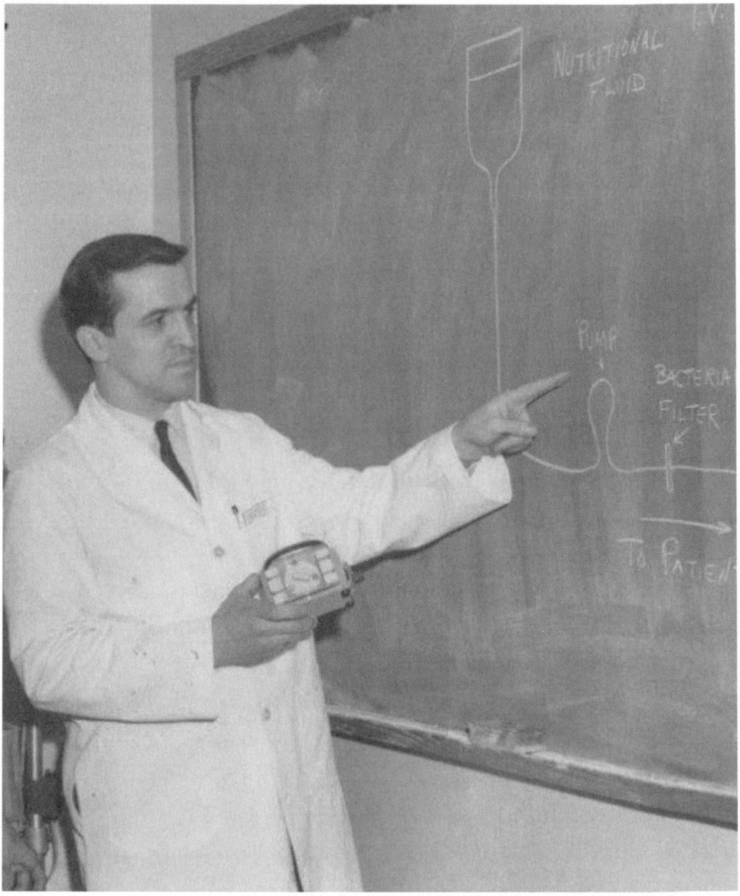

Stanley J. Dudrick, MD, 1973.

An important part of improving the emergency room and critical care service was working closely with the nursing staff. As the critical care service began to grow, Dudrick proposed a plan to the hospital and to the nurses for developing a specialized critical-care nursing service that included nurses from the emergency room, the medical intensive care unit, the surgical intensive care unit, the anesthesia preoperative unit, the post-anesthesia immediate care unit, and the operating room. Nursing administrators approved the plan, and these nurses formed a group that made up the core of critical-care nurses. "We got one of the best nurses in the hospital to become head of the critical-care nursing unit, and they started rotating them around," said Dudrick. "It improved morale. It improved care. It was an innovation that evolved out of need and wanting to satisfy the need."[7]

In addition to improving relations with the first responders and establishing a critical-care nursing team, the surgeons also saw the need to bring more of the medical school's faculty, interns, and residents in to help, as the number of emergency room patients began to grow. They also wanted to have more specialists available to provide treatment. "We were going through a period of evolution," said Red Duke of those early days. "When we started this thing, we decided that we were going to take over the emergency room—we were going to run a trauma service and a surgical service. And for a while, only the surgical service ran the ER. And then, we gradually enticed the internists to put their residents down there." Eduardo Souchon, one of the surgical residents, recalled, "The beginning was extremely hard. There were two services for Trauma—Dudrick's and Duke's service. So, the residents were divided in two and we took call every other night." Within a few months, they established a small area in the back of the emergency room to provide pediatric care. Thus, with the UT doctors taking on more of the trauma care responsibilities in the emergency service, most of the old house staff gradually left the ER to attend to other duties in the hospital.[8]

But at this time, the population and resultant traffic congestion in Houston and the surrounding region was growing dramatically, and there were only a few hospitals capable of providing comprehensive specialty care to seriously injured or ill patients. Recognizing this issue, Stan Dudrick, Red Duke, and EMS Chief Lester "Whitey" Martin approached William "Bill" Smith, CEO of Hermann Hospital, with a proposal to start a civilian air medical program capable of quickly transporting critically injured or seriously ill patients from distant hospitals or accident locations to Hermann Hospital. Prior to this, in 1973, Houston businessman and philanthropist John S. Dunn took the first step in making this air ambulance service a reality when he donated the funds to build a helistop at Hermann Hospital. Dan G. Kadrovach, who at the time was director (CEO) of Hermann Hospital, was a strong supporter of the helicopter service. Kadrovach, who had been appointed director in 1966,

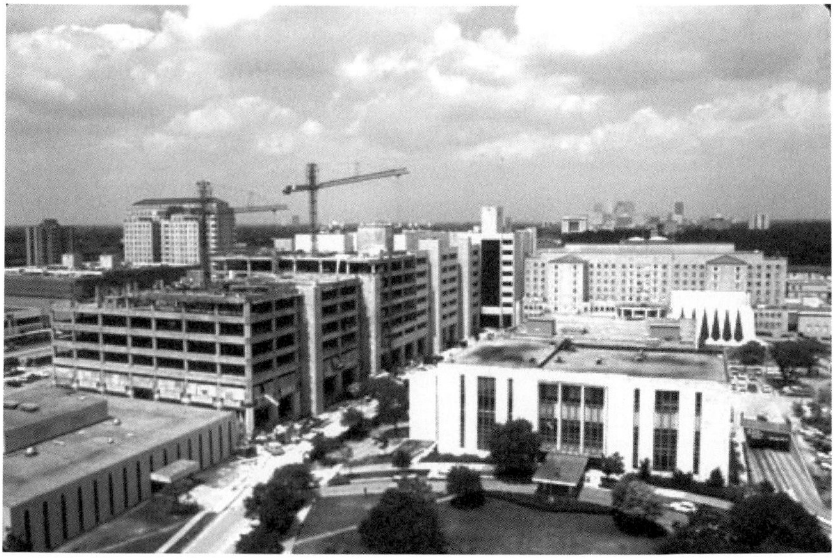

Main Medical School Building under construction, 1975. Freeman Building is front left, Hermann Hospital center rear, and Jesse H. Jones Building, Texas Medical Center Library in foreground.

had served in the army in Germany as a medical service officer and was familiar with the benefits of fast evacuation military medicine as it was used in Vietnam, along with the value of helicopters rapidly transporting seriously wounded soldiers to medical facilities. As Cheves Smythe recalled, until he was replaced by Bill Smith in 1976, Kadrovach was the unquestioning support person regarding helicopter evacuation and was "an enthusiastic supporter of the emergence of what the surgeons were doing. To have the hospital director on your side really helps," said Smythe. John Dunn was one of the Hermann Estate trustees, the board that ran the hospital. The John S. Dunn Helistop opened in 1973, providing Houston and the surrounding area with the first medical helicopter facility in the Texas Medical Center since the failed landing pad operated by Airlift Inc. more than twenty years earlier. It is important here to note that a heliport, a helistop, and a helipad are three different things. A helipad is just a pad where a helicopter can land. By contrast, a helistop has lights and can provide minimal service to the helicopter, while a heliport must offer full service, including fueling and mechanical support. Helipad, helistop, and heliport, then, are graduated levels of service. Stanley Dudrick recalled that initially, the trustees wanted to build the helistop on the ground, next to the emergency room entrance. He convinced Dunn that the hospital would be better served, for safety and security reasons, if the helistop was built on the second-floor level. "I told them that our ground space was the most precious commodity in that Medical Center," said Dudrick. "That is why that helistop was built on the second floor but then, of course, we had to put in an elevator so that it could go down one floor to the emergency room." This met some opposition, but in the end, Dudrick was able to convince Dunn and the trustees.[9]

By the mid-1970s, with construction of the main medical school building underway, Hermann Hospital also began work on a new building that would be contiguous with the medical school, known in time as the Jones Pavilion. Among the features on the drawing board were new operating rooms. Much of the design had been completed during the planning stage before Dudrick joined the medical school. As he reviewed the plans for the new operating rooms, he was dismayed by what he saw. Over the years, as he traveled the country, Dudrick had many opportunities to visit hospitals and see the latest innovations for operating rooms. After trying to work with the architects to make the new Hermann Hospital facility meet the standards of a modern operating room, he convinced the architect that they needed to start over. They began to redesign the operating rooms, reducing the number to provide more space in those that would remain. Dudrick also had a temporary model built outside the hospital, in which the surgeons could view the latest equipment and have input into the design. This allowed the surgical staff to see the equipment in place and visualize how it might work. It also gave everyone the opportunity to have some input and reach a general consensus. When the new Jones Pavilion opened in 1977, it had "the best operating rooms in Houston," said Dudrick. "We did a lot to try to make things work. It did not just happen. I had a significant investment of my life—blood, sweat, and tears—in the place, and I think we gave it a fantastic start." With a newly enhanced emergency room and first-rate, modern operating rooms, Hermann Hospital was poised to move into a new era of trauma care.[10]

Dudrick continued to push for developing the helicopter service but still met resistance from some staff and trustees who worried about the cost. He urged patience and encouraged the doubters to view investment in the project as they would any business proposition. It would take time for the helicopter to bring a return. "The people who did not like it were never going to like it," said Dudrick. "And the people who liked it were going to, no matter what, but we were the ones that were pushing it. I was not wise enough to foresee how important that helicopter was going to be down the line, but I got wise as I saw what was happening."[11]

By 1976, with the helistop open at Hermann Hospital, the idea for creating a helicopter ambulance service had time to germinate and gain some momentum. Dudrick and Duke had some initial ideas of their own and also did extensive research to learn from existing programs. In fact, only a few hospitals offered landing pads for helicopters. The first civilian and hospital-based air ambulance service in the United States was the St. Anthony Central Hospital's "Flight for Life" in Denver, which began service in 1972. Duke recalled that EMS Chief Lester "Whitey" Martin had learned about the Denver-based Flight for Life at a meeting. Shortly, representatives from Houston visited the hospital in Denver to learn more about the helicopter service. Red Duke later recalled that while the group in Denver did not exactly roll out the red carpet to welcome the delegation from Houston, the group still learned a lot about types of equipment and the mechanics of making a helicopter ambulance service work. Armed with this knowledge and the ideas they had been working through, Duke, Dudrick, and Whitey Martin convinced Hermann Hospital's CEO, Bill Smith, to support the project. After their visit to Denver to see the service at St. Anthony's, they fleshed out the plan, enabling Smith to convince the hospital's board of trustees to provide operating funds to lease a helicopter, pilots, and a mechanic for six months.[12]

One of the lasting impressions they took back to Houston was the utility of the French Alouette helicopter, which was equipped with high-powered engines designed to fly in the thin air of the French Alps. "It is a French helicopter made for mountain rescue in Switzerland and France," said Duke. "And it was interesting, the patients were side-loaded like bread into an oven behind the pilot, and the guy on the top had better not be very sick, because they did not have any access to him." The hospital leased the Alouette from Rocky Mountain Helicopters, which also provided the pilots and mechanics.[13]

Once the helicopter ambulance was approved, Dudrick and Duke quickly had to learn the intricate details of how to operate such a service. How should they staff the helicopter? What training would the flight crew need? Protocols had to be developed for everything, including how to identify safe landing zones (LZs). And with so much going on simultaneously in the Department of Surgery, Dudrick realized it was time to delegate responsibility for some of the department's activities. "When Jim Duke came, I asked him to look after trauma," said Dudrick. "I asked Ted Copeland to look after cancer, and I thought I would take care of the rest." As department chair, Dudrick had administrative and supervisory responsibilities over all of the department's divisions and was fortunate to have Duke and Copeland to take the lead in these demanding areas. Ted Copeland remembered the hectic pace of those days: "Red and Stan were both involved in setting up the helicopter transport system," said Copeland. "It was one of the first in the United States, as a matter of fact."[14]

Next was to determine how to staff the helicopter. They needed trained flight nurses as part of the crew, but as Red Duke recalled, there was no manual, no "recipe" for how to train them. "We had to figure out how we were going to do this," said Duke, "so we chose several really good ICU nurses and some ER nurses, and we conducted our education program there in the emergency room." They taught the nurses how to intubate, how to recognize vital signs, and how to give certain medications in the field. "I wanted to make sure that we put the best possible teams on the helicopter," said Dudrick. "And we had either an intern or a first-year resident on the flights for the first few years. It was exciting to them, and they loved to do it." The doctors on board the helicopter communicated with the hospital by headset and radio. When they arrived at the scene, they provided immediate medical care that included everything from starting IVs, intubating patients, resuscitating them, cardiac massage, or whatever needed to be done. They would stop any bleeding, apply splints, protect patients' necks, and get them on the helicopter and on the way to Hermann Hospital. Eduardo Souchon was one of the residents who made up those early helicopter crews. "In the beginning, we were flight doctors," said Souchon. "We would go in the helicopter with a nurse and a pilot, retrieve the injured, and bring them here. It was fun and it was fascinating. It was like *M*A*S*H.*" As Souchon observed, Hermann Hospital quickly became a true trauma hospital and in 1990, was designated as the area's first Level I Trauma Center. Today, Memorial Hermann–TMC is known as one of the busiest trauma centers in the world.[15]

The helicopter arrived in May 1976. "We had three months to get this thing put together," said Red Duke. "We had already done a lot of work before we got to that point. We had the nurses pretty well trained. They were pioneers—you've got to admire them. On August 1, 1976, we took a deep breath and started. That first day we made three flights, and forty-five the first month, and it just kept on." In the beginning, then, the flight crews consisted of a pilot, a nurse, and physician. The dramatic sight of a helicopter landing at Hermann Hospital quickly became a popular feature for local television news. Because the helicopter flew on a mission almost every day, the television coverage amounted to free publicity. Soon, Drs. Duke and Dudrick began to notice a steadily increasing number of walk-in patients in the emergency room. Dudrick stated that when asked why they were coming to Hermann, patients often replied that they had seen the helicopter on television and concluded it must be the best place to go for emergency treatment. "We never counted on that, but it happened," said Dudrick. "We started filling the hospital up. We started getting overwhelmed and before you knew it, we needed a second helicopter and, you know, it just grew." Eventually, the surgical interns and residents stopped flying on Life Flight, replaced by trained Emergency Medical Technicians (EMT) and nurses with advanced, specialized training. Hermann Hospital was growing in size and patient load, and it was more cost-effective and efficient to have the physicians remain on duty at the hospital.[16]

One of the ongoing aspects of the first year of Life Flight was the continuing need to develop protocols for the many situations the helicopter and crew might encounter, from daily operations to the exigencies. Drs. Red Duke and William P. Clarke, along with the head nurse and the chief pilot, met regularly, usually in the early morning at a little semi-private side room in the hospital cafeteria, where they wrote protocols for everything including flight crews, medication, and safety on the landing pad. One of the most important issues they addressed was landing zones. Sometimes, the helicopter would pick up a critically injured patient at another hospital to bring them back to Hermann. But in those days, hospitals did not have helipads or established landing zones. "We did not have any landing zones anywhere," said Red Duke. "When we would go to a hospital, it was usually a parking lot that we would land in. And many times, these were just gravel parking lots." The force of air from the helicopter blades sent gravel and sand flying, often damaging nearby parked cars. "We had to pay for a bunch of paint jobs on cars, because they got sanded pretty well," said Duke. "And one of the things we started doing was conducting training programs on how to build heliports." They also began training local EMS teams how to find a safe landing zone on locations away from a hospital. "There were certain criteria—lighting, and you had to worry about trees and power lines, particularly at night," said Duke. "On an EMS call, you've got to go wherever they are." In the beginning, Life Flight was considered to be an experiment, and the hospital did not provide very much in the way of communications infrastructure to support the program. "Our communication system was a red telephone on the triage desk," said Duke. He recalled doing a lot of public relations work during those first months, particularly with the Harris County Medical Society, all in an effort to encourage EMS to bring more patients to Hermann Hospital. The UT surgeons saw this not as a matter of competition with Ben Taub Hospital, but as a practical matter, since there were many emergency cases in the city. With a growing patient population, the Hermann Hospital Estate allocated an additional six months of funds for the helicopter service, which officially adopted the name Life Flight, and appointed Red Duke as Medical Director for the program.[17]

A few months later, just before 8:00 a.m. on St. Patrick's Day, March 17, 1977, the main stabilizer unit at the Texaco refinery in nearby Port Arthur, Texas, exploded, when what was described as a "fog" of flammable gas escaped and ignited into flames. The ensuing fire injured twenty-two workers, with seventeen sustaining critical burns, and caused extensive damage to the 150 foot–high stabilizer unit. According to news reports, immediately after the blast, survivors rushed to the unit, dragged their injured comrades to safety, and began to fight the fire. The company's firefighters brought the blaze under control and had it extinguished by noon. The injured first were transported to St. Mary's Hospital in Port Arthur, where doctors quickly determined that the most seriously burned needed more attention. They notified Hermann Hospital and John Sealy Hospital in Galveston that they had several who were critically burned, including one man burned over 97 percent of his body, and several others burned over 61 to 80 percent of their bodies. Life Flight was called to bring some of the severely injured and burned patients to Hermann Hospital. Helicopters from army medical detachments at Fort Polk, Louisiana, and from the Military Assistance for Safety and Traffic (MAST), a reserve unit at Tomball, also brought patients, with a total of ten victims coming to Hermann and six going to John Sealy Hospital in Galveston, where five less seriously injured patients also arrived by ambulance. In addition, the Houston Fire Department and Ben Taub Hospital also played key roles in the airlift of the critically injured to major burn centers.[18]

"We did not have a real burn unit, but Jim and I knew how to take care of burns," said Dudrick. He mobilized the nurses and housekeeping to help assemble a stockpile of towels, bed sheets, bandages, and IV fluids. They prepared several rooms to provide the special care required for burn patients. Dudrick had put out a call, and soon all available medical staff and students reported to the emergency room, ready to help. "We were ready for them," said Dudrick years later. "We were ready for fifty." Local television stations covered the arrival of Life Flight and the army helicopters with TV cameras and reporters, while other members of the press took photographs and wrote up their stories. "We started hauling in burn victims, and we had all kinds of TV cameras and press downstairs," said Duke. "With all that attention, it is amazing how many people really became big supporters [of the helicopter ambulance]. Maybe it wasn't as crazy as it sounded. We got great press, and people care about that ... free advertising." At the time, Hermann did not have the capability to provide care for more than six burn patients at a time on a long-term basis. As a result, on the Saturday following the explosion, officials arranged for two of the less critically injured patients at Hermann to be flown to Brooke Army Hospital in San Antonio, and two more went to

Parkland Hospital in Dallas. Five of the injured remained at Hermann, and six other victims were in critical condition in John Sealy Hospital in Galveston. Sadly, seventeen of the twenty-two who were burned in the blast eventually died of their injuries.[19]

In the aftermath, the quick response by the helicopter team and the positive television coverage helped convince the last skeptics of the merits of Life Flight. Dudrick recalled that Texaco gave Hermann Hospital a commendation for the superb emergency response and patient care and also provided some of the seed money to build an initial Burn Unit at the hospital. Soon the medical school brought in Dr. Donald H. Parks, a plastic surgeon, as burn director. "We got that burn unit started and that was kind of a fringe benefit of the helicopter, and our willingness to meet the needs of the community, which I thought was our primary goal," said Dudrick. "And from that moment on, we started getting a fair share of the trauma patients from the ambulances, in addition to the helicopter."[20]

During the years since Life Flight first began in Houston, dozens of other helicopter services arose across the country. Many of them sent representatives to Houston to learn from the Life Flight team. Some of the country's most renowned surgeons also came to visit, to see for themselves how the program worked. As Dudrick recalled, "We gave talks about it and they often copied what we did." Dudrick's mentor and former boss, Dr. Jonathan Rhoads from the University of Pennsylvania, was one of the visitors. "We gave him a ride in the helicopter and showed him what we were doing," said Dudrick. "People were fascinated. Dr. Francis Moore, who was the father of metabolic surgery at Harvard, came down as our visiting professor—he wanted to see that helicopter. So, that was clearly a major advance in medicine in the country." Dudrick believed that lessons from the Vietnam War helped encourage the development of the civilian air ambulance services. Early evacuation improved outcomes. "We applied directly what we learned in Vietnam to civilian practice in a huge metropolitan radius with log-jam traffic and distances to overcome," stated Dudrick. "If you could not get people into the operating room within one hour from the time they were hurt, your chances of saving them dropped geometrically. So, it was an application of it." A second Alouette was added to the fleet in 1977, and it expanded once again in 1978 to include a third Alouette. All three aircraft were based at Hermann Hospital, assigned flights on a rotating basis and dispatched from offices below the helistop. At that time, the service area extended 120 miles from Hermann Hospital.[21]

The growing success of trauma care at the Medical School was closely tied to the contributions of divisions within the Department of Surgery. These included Emergency General, Oral and Maxillofacial, and Plastic and Reconstructive. Working out of the ICU, critical-care surgeons from the division of Emergency General Surgery addressed cases including bowel obstruction, appendicitis, burns, and any others that required urgent or immediate care. Oral and Maxillofacial Surgery and Plastic and Reconstructive Surgery were also integral to Acute Care. While their primary importance resided with the dental school, oral and maxillofacial surgeons and residents provided dependable, quality care to patients suffering head, neck, and facial injuries. Dr. Frank Moody, who would succeed Stan Dudrick as department chair in 1982, remembered them fondly: "We had a lot of interaction with the dental residents, and they were very bright. But what I liked about them is they would crack jokes and were a lot of fun." By the late 1970s, the fundamental involvement of the dental surgeons to both acute and general surgery sparked a program in oral and maxillofacial surgery that had become part of the surgical residency.[22]

The division of Plastic and Reconstructive Surgery also played an important role. Up to three plastic surgeons comprised a team focusing upon trauma reconstruction, the treatment of serious burns, and reconstruction of burn tissue. Their efforts were enhanced by the development of a major, comprehensive burn center at Hermann. Funded through the John S. Dunn Foundation, a local nonprofit organization dedicated to the support of medical care and research, the center began operations in the late 1970s, and until recently, was directed by the UT Division of Plastic Surgery. The development of the Burn Center at Hermann over the past four decades is a source of great pride to the UT faculty surgeons. "It is really hard work, and it never was that easy to recruit individuals to do major trauma," observed UT plastic surgeon Donald H. Parks. However, the center's effectiveness not only provided the Medical School plastic surgeons an exciting and interesting arena, but gave the department a foundation for growth.[23]

Along with these aspects of surgery, Stan Dudrick also had recruited faculty who had an interest in nutrition. Several of the team went on to great success in this area during the 1970s and beyond. At M. D. Anderson Cancer Center, Ted Copeland applied total parenteral nutrition (TPN) to cancer patients, something that had never been done before. His work in this area made him well known around the country. Copeland had been an army doctor in Vietnam and used TPN on patients there. He applied the same principles of nutrition to cancer patients at M. D. Anderson. Bruce MacFadyen, the first resident to come with Dudrick from the University of Pennsylvania, worked closely for a year with Copeland at M. D. Anderson. At the time, there were two major concerns related to using TPN on cancer patients: first, that the indwelling catheters would create a locus for infection in people who, because they were being treated with chemotherapy and radiation therapy, had low white counts; and second, that the nutritive therapy itself would make the cancers grow. "We encountered a group of people over there who were so malnourished that they could not be treated absent intravenous nutrition," said Copeland. "They could not eat. No choice. So, I had no problem with the institution on whether I could begin to use TPN in those people." M. D. Anderson's nurses helped with TPN by providing excellent patient care with special attention to the catheters. The infection rates were extremely low, and the tumors did not grow. Soon Copeland and MacFadyen were publishing papers in the medical journals and also becoming known for their work around the country. Copeland became nationally renowned for using TPN in cancer patients. In time, they started a home TPN service for cancer patients. In addition to TPN, they also pioneered new cancer surgery and treatments. "We were one of the first to do lumpectomies," said Copeland. "We were the first to use radiation therapy on large cancers of the rectum and shrink them down and not have to do colostomies." This work contributed to a database that, as Copeland explained, "was a gold mine for anybody who had any real interest in academic research."[24]

In the late 1970s, the American Medical Association asked Bruce MacFadyen to do a presentation on the use of total parenteral nutrition and some of the complications that they had seen, based on a paper he and Copeland had written on the metabolic problems and solutions of

TPN. As part of the research, MacFadyen decided to look back on what they had done at the Medical School over the last year. He was amazed to find that during that time, they had treated over 1,000 patients with total parenteral nutrition, far above the numbers anywhere else. The UT team had very low infection rates, in part because they had established a nutrition team that would monitor patients and change the dressings. "We were very particular," said MacFadyen. As a result, he noted, "We had very, very low complication rates, low infection rates." After he completed his residency, MacFadyen spent the next year at M. D. Anderson working with Ted Copeland. He noted that even among cancer patients, a group at high risk for infection, they had a very low complication rate. They had developed a nutrition team that included nurses, nutritionists, and fellows. In time, people came from around the world to M. D. Anderson to learn about total parenteral nutrition and to see for themselves how the UT team was organized.[25]

Soon, Copeland and MacFadyen were also doing more presentations. Even places as esteemed as Massachusetts General and Harvard were just starting TPN programs. "It was really an exciting time, because it was very new and it was very useful," said MacFadyen. Many patients survived multiple complications. Prior to the use of TPN, clinical results showed a mortality rate of 40 to 60 percent. But with the use of intravenous nutrition, the mortality dropped to about 5 percent. Patients were surviving major operations because their bodies were getting the nutrition needed to sustain them and fight infections. "Very few people were doing it [TPN] at that time," said MacFadyen. "It was fun being in on the ground floor of that whole process. That is how the TPN got started. That is how the whole department grew."[26]

Ted Copeland reflected on the excitement of the early days and how it shaped his career. "I owe my career to UT-Houston as well as M. D. Anderson," said Copeland. "I had the best job that will ever exist in academic surgery." Copeland gratefully acknowledged how Red Duke took call in the emergency room so he could continue his work at M. D. Anderson. "God knows why he did that, but he did, without ever complaining, and any time I complained he said, 'Forget it. Go over there and work. You are doing great stuff.'" In 1982, Copeland left Houston for Gainesville, Florida, where he continued a stellar career as Professor and Chairman of the Department of Surgery at the University of Florida College of Medicine.[27]

Other divisions put their own stamp upon the Medical School's surgical program. One such division was Pediatric Surgery. The groundbreaking pediatric surgeon, Benjy Brooks, was an early star on Dudrick's team. Described as a "character" by those who knew her, Brooks, a Texas native, shouldered her way through a difficult, male-dominated field to become the first female pediatric surgeon in America. A 1948 graduate of The University of Texas Medical Branch, Brooks accepted residencies at medical centers in Pennsylvania and Boston before arriving at the Texas Medical Center in 1958. Once in Houston, Brooks joined the surgical team at Texas Children's Hospital, while giving additional hours to patients at St. Joseph's Hospital. Her daily routine was rewarding yet emotionally difficult. Occasionally, the demands of operating on "broken babies" on a daily basis compelled Brooks to drive to a local playground to watch children at play. "That was one of the ways I built my morale, to know that there were children that were laughing and running and playing in the world."[28]

By the early 1970s, The University of Texas Medical School at Houston needed a pediatric surgeon on the medical school faculty. Although her career had been devoted to private practice, Brooks was an attractive draw. In 1973, Dudrick invited Brooks aboard as division director of pediatric surgery, a position she held until her retirement in 1982. Outspoken, energetic, and independent, Brooks became an institution in her own right during her years at UT-Houston. She established an innovative surgical program, loved mentoring, and was a role model for many an admiring medical student. Performing delicate procedures on at-risk infants became a specialty. By the end of her surgical career, Brooks had supervised more than 20,000 surgeries on infants, some weighing less than two pounds. In addition to a rigorous teaching and surgical schedule, Brooks maintained productive lines of research that included congenital defects, the treatment of burns, and the prevention of hepatitis.[29] It has been more than thirty years since Benjy Brooks retired from practice. Yet her legacy continues to be felt at the medical school. Inspired by her young patients, Brooks established the Benjy Brooks Foundation for Children, a nonprofit organization dedicated to the advancement

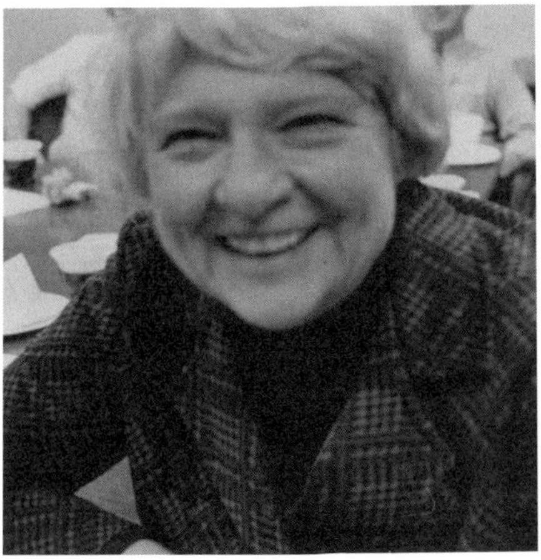

Benjy F. Brooks, MD.

of pediatric surgical care in Texas. Moreover, the Benjy Brooks Library, located inside the UT-Houston complex, is a valuable repository for pediatric resources and materials. In 1985, Dr. Richard J. Andrassy stepped into Brooks's role as division chair of Pediatric Surgery. In this capacity, Andrassy effectively maintained the vibrancy of the Brooks years while continuing to develop a reputation for clinical and academic excellence.

The young faculty of the Department of Surgery not only proved to be hardworking, dedicated surgeons, but also prolific scholars. "I think the first two years that we were here in Houston, the Department of Surgery produced more than 50 or 60 papers," said Dudrick. "For a brand new school that did not even have formal laboratories at that time, we produced a lot of research." They worked closely with other departments, including Physiology, and with the Radiation Department and many of the oncologists at M. D. Anderson. These collaborative efforts were useful and mutually beneficial to the other departments. They developed a department of surgery that was unique in that every member that was recruited had an interest in nutrition and metabolic support of patients in addition to his or her primary specialty. "That was a first," said Dudrick. "There was no department that had ever done that before . . . no other group that I know of ever had accomplished that. I thought that we produced the finest general surgery division in the city." Indeed, The University of Texas Medical School's Department of Surgery created its own niche in Houston, a community where M. D. Anderson was cancer-based and the Texas Heart Institute and Baylor College of Medicine both were cardiovascular and vascular-based. But at that time, there was no real home for general surgery in Houston. As Dudrick noted, UT's initial group of four pioneering surgeons created a first-rate, physiologically and biochemically based general surgery department right in the heart of the Texas Medical Center.[30]

In addition to developing an increasingly renowned department of surgery, The University of Texas Medical School at Houston, in time and with the help of Dr. Denton Cooley, was able to launch a cardiovascular service, literally in the backyard of Baylor College of Medicine and famed heart surgeon Dr. Michael DeBakey. Cooley's help added prestige and attracted residents to the program, especially when he agreed to take UT students and residents at the Texas Heart Institute. "He was very good to us," said Dudrick. "Operating room #7 at the Texas Heart Institute was always manned, so to speak, by University of Texas students and residents and supervised by Dr. Cooley and his faculty." All of this brought an air of excitement for residents who relished the opportunity to work with Denton Cooley's team. They wanted to be part of the Texas Heart Institute, which, as Dudrick observed, "is still kind of magical in the hearts and minds of Houstonians and Texans."[31]

Other milestones included starting the first home ambulatory nutrition and metabolic center in the country. This expanded into home care, sending patients home on intravenous feeding who otherwise did not need to remain in the hospital. In time the unit grew into a profitable concern and was sold to Home Health Care of America. But as Dudrick recalled, "The reason we started the home care was at one point in time, I had thirty-six patients at Hermann Hospital, and the only reason they were there was they were getting intravenous feeding. We could send them home, but there was nobody to take care of them at home. So, we started this unit where we could get them out of the hospital so they could have a more normal life and yet come back to this unit to be serviced; or we could send people out from the unit to take care of them within a certain radius." They also got into support of athletics, working with Houston professional sports teams including the Astros, Rockets, and the Oilers in promoting fitness and nutritional support. They worked behind the scenes with NASA to help develop better oral diets for the astronauts and to try to package high-potency supplements for them. Dudrick noted that after starting those early ventures in metabolism, nutrition, and physiology in 1972, forty years later, the world is now doing what they talked about back then. "For me, it is like a dream come true," said Dudrick. "We still have an enormous voyage for the future, but I think I can stand proudly with the faculty and the students and the residents and the fellows and the other supporters of The University of Texas Health Science Center and say that we really did our part. It did not just happen."[32]

All of this growth and success ultimately led to one of the faculty becoming something of a television star. When construction on Phase II of the main building began in September 1973, one of the components was a small television studio designed for educational film production including a health series entitled *Texas Health Letter* that also could be broadcast on public or commercial television. "They didn't have any money to hire a professional, so they asked me if I would try it," said Red Duke. "I didn't know anything about TV and still don't. We did four of them the next year, and nobody ever showed them." But one thing led to another and in time, Houston television station KTRK–Channel 13 aired one of the broadcasts. Duke later admitted that he was not quite sure how to end his segment, so he simply stated, "From The University of Texas Health Science Center in Houston, I'm Dr. Red Duke," which became his trademark sign-off. Channel 13 wanted more of the show, and soon word spread about the folksy Houston doctor and his health series. In time, it was syndicated to some seventy-three television stations, picked up by the Armed Forces Network, and aired for about fifteen years. The program, known by various titles, including *Dr. Red Duke's Health Reports*, brought public attention to the UT Medical School and a measure of fame to Red Duke. But what Duke cared most about was treating patients, not being a TV star. "All I knew how to do was work, and that is all I want to do," said Duke. "I really love it—taking care of patients. It is such an honor to have the responsibility of being a physician. There is no profession to equal it, because the responsibility is enormous. The privilege of being able to do these things is beyond words."[33]

The 1970s truly were booming years for the Department of Surgery. By the end of the decade, the department was thriving, providing a high level of patient care, developing new and better ways to treat trauma patients, and leading the way in research on total parenteral nutrition. The Life Flight, done in conjunction with Hermann Hospital, proved to be a great success. It brought favorable publicity to the hospital, to the UT-Houston Medical School, and to the department of surgery. Dr. Phillip R. Adams, who first arrived as a medical student in 1973, has witnessed the degree of change over time. "The trauma service began growing when the helicopter was put in when I was an intern," said Adams. "That grew the program dramatically. And subsequently, the hospital caught up over time with their facilities and also, in the tradition of the Texas Medical Center, it got bigger and better. Our ability to care for the critically ill patient has changed dramatically over the years and improved dramatically. I am proud to be part of that."[34]

In reflecting back on those early years of the department, Dudrick concluded: "It took courage to think that we could come down as a group of young people and start a medical school and do as well or better than many other schools that had had distinguished, long-term faculty for years and had the depth of support and acres of laboratory space and millions of dollars; and yet, we were able to put out a product that was equal to or better than many other institutions."[35]

But with all of the success came many distractions for Dudrick. His busy schedule and frequent travel left little time for the intricacies and politics of departmental administration. The growing prominence of the department of surgery and particularly its chairman also engendered criticism and perhaps a level of professional envy. As the decade of the 1970s drew to a close, high-level administrative changes at The University of Texas Health Science Center soon would have drastic implications for Stan Dudrick, the Department of Surgery, and the entire University of Texas Medical School.

CHAPTER 4

The Transplant Era

During the first ten years of its history, The University of Texas Medical School at Houston achieved great success but also endured a series of administrative changes that at times shocked the school, created unwelcome publicity, and eventually touched the Department of Surgery. In 1972, UT had created The University of Texas Health Science Center–Houston as an organizational structure that encompassed all of the university's Houston medical schools except the M. D. Anderson Cancer Center, naming Dr. John V. Olson, dean of the UT Dental Branch, as acting president. In December 1974, the university appointed Dr. Charles Berry, who had been director of medical programs at NASA, as president. Just three months later, Berry fired Cheves M. Smythe from his position as dean of the medical school. Dr. Robert L. Tuttle was named interim dean and in December officially became the second dean of the medical school. The revolving door continued to turn, and in February 1977, Charles A. Berry resigned his post as the first president of the UT Health Science Center. Truman G. Blocker Jr., MD, president emeritus of The University of Texas Medical Branch at Galveston, was invited to come to UT-Houston as acting president. Blocker was a large man of prominent girth, described as a dynamic physician with an infectious inquiry who possessed a handshake that "could bring tears to your eyes." From his remodeled offices in the Freeman Building, Blocker remained in close proximity to the Medical School faculty and projects—including the first organ transplants. As acting president of the UT Health Science Center, Blocker created the tradition of annually awarding the Gold-Headed Cane to an outstanding student in medicine and ethics.[1]

Blocker's vibrant oversight of UT-Houston continued until the early summer of 1978. In June, Roger Bulger, MD became the second president of the Health Science Center. Determined to instigate change where he deemed necessary, Bulger set his sights upon the administrative workings of each department—surgery in particular. While Bulger was put off by Dudrick's popularity and power within the medical school, the primary issues were administrative. Brilliance in teaching and research does not necessarily transfer to executive talent. As surgery chair, Dudrick actively utilized his fame and political expertise to acquire funding, faculty, and other necessities for departmental growth. Yet daily tasks and political challenges of administrative work were often overlooked, in part due to Dudrick's heavy travel schedule. "Stan was this international figure by this time and flew all over the world giving talks, which was part of the problem," Joseph Corriere recalled of this period. "Stan tried to run the department with a telephone and an airplane." As a result, the surgery department found itself deeply in debt by the end of its first decade, indicating that there had been little scrutiny or protest from the dean's office.[2]

As the second dean of the medical school, Bob Tuttle was well liked but non-confrontational. "Bob was the nicest guy in the world who could not say no" remembered Corriere. Tuttle undoubtedly hesitated to dampen the collegial environment and professional acclaim Dudrick had created for the medical school. "Dr. Dudrick was such a personable person," Richard Andrassy noted of this period, "I mean, he was just larger than life, having developed TPN." In the minds of many faculty and staff, Dudrick's leadership was instrumental to the high reputation UT surgeons held in the national and international medical community.[3]

President Bulger thought otherwise. In the months following Bulger's arrival, tensions mounted as he and Dudrick continued to experience incompatibilities. In August of 1980—after two years of conflict with the president's office—Dudrick resigned the surgery chairmanship. "It was obvious to me that Dr. Bulger and I were never going to see eye-to-eye," said Dudrick years later. "If I did not agree not to seek a renewal on my contract, I had a feeling that it would just be a matter of time until he would conjure up some reason to fire me. . . .There was a lot of turmoil about it. People could not understand why I did not fight him more and all that, but it would have been a mess." The news created a terrific flap on the medical school campus. Not only was Dudrick stepping down, but also word got out that President Bulger had also removed the highly respected pathology chairman, Donald C. Cannon. Rumors began to spread involving other senior faculty being forced to step aside. While these tales were unfounded, some within the medical school began to fear a major faculty shake-up. By August 5, more than fifty Medical School faculty, residents, and students signed a petition protesting the removals. The turmoil continued throughout the fall of 1980, as a highly publicized threat of a lawsuit by Cannon and several faculty captured local newspaper headlines, providing the medical school weeks of unwanted publicity.[4]

By early November, the UT regents had seen enough. While partially critical of Bulger's administrative management, members of the board joined UT System Chancellor E. Don Walker in providing an unusual public vote of confidence to Bulger. Disgruntled faculty and residents in surgery and pathology were urged to accept the administrative changes within their respective departments. In the end, both Dudrick and Cannon remained as full professors at the medical school. Indeed, Dudrick was far from gone. Having been the youngest chief of surgery at an American medical college when he came to Houston in 1972, Dudrick relinquished his post at the still-vibrant age of 45. And there was still much to do. "I actually got the biggest raise I ever got in my life for the next year, and that had to go across [Bulger's] desk," Dudrick later recalled. "I do not know who engineered it . . . but I just kept doing what I was doing, except being chairman. There were some uncomfortable times, and I felt more sorry for other people's discomfort than my own . . . It was not the end of the world." Over the next fourteen years, from 1980 to 1994, Dudrick remained on the faculty, except for a brief return to Philadelphia in beginning in 1988, where he joined the staff of Pennsylvania Hospital as Chairman of the Department of Surgery, Surgeon to the Hospital, Director of the Residency Training Program in General Surgery, and Clinical Professor of Surgery at the University of Pennsylvania. Dudrick returned to Houston on May 1, 1990, when he was appointed Surgeon-in-Chief of the Center for Cardiovascular Disease and Director of the Hermann Nutrition and Human Performance Center, the Nutritional Support Service, and the Nutritional Science Center at Hermann Hospital, and Clinical Professor of Surgery at The University of Texas Medical School at Houston. He left Houston for good, late in 1994, for Waterbury, Connecticut, where he accepted an appointment as Associate

Chairman of the Department of Surgery at Saint Mary's Hospital and as Professor of Surgery at Yale University School of Medicine. In October 2007, Dudrick became Chairman Emeritus, Department of Surgery.[5]

In the meantime, the surgery chairmanship was delegated elsewhere. Appointed by Dean Tuttle as interim chair, Joseph Corriere faced the burden of untangling various knots within the department while a search committee investigated a full-time hire. Although Corriere did not relish the prospect of administrative work—especially that of an acting chair—he was well suited for the task. Having already developed a strong academic program in urology and at that time president of the UT Medical School's Faculty Senate, Corriere understood the development of management systems and the financial requirements to sustain them. "Joe really knew the inside workings of things," Andrassy later noted. [6]

The first thing on Corriere's docket was the creation of a new budget. "What I tried to do was look at where all the money was going and see what we could stop," he remembered, "We tried canceling all sorts of things." He voided outstanding orders for furniture and equipment and whittled departmental staff, firing almost twenty-five lab technicians and administrative assistants. The most difficult task, however, was letting go of faculty. "That is where a lot of money is, in salaries," Corriere reasoned, "So . . . we had to close down some areas . . . The hard part for me was, not only did I have to get rid of faculty, but I also had to recruit some faculty." Dr. Thomas A. Miller, a general surgeon well trained in gastrointestinal (GI) diseases, was put in charge of the residency program. The trauma unit and helicopter service was expanding rapidly at Hermann Hospital, requiring new hires. Corriere considered himself "lucky" to acquire Dr. Ronald P. Fischer, a general surgeon and Chair of Surgery at the University of Arizona Medical School in Tucson, to oversee the endeavor. A Vietnam veteran, Fischer received a Bronze Star in 1968 for his service as Chief of Surgery at the Saigon 3rd Army Field Hospital. "Those guys who had done one year [in Vietnam] really were great surgeons," Corriere noted. "They really understood trauma. [Fischer] came in and ran the trauma service for a long time . . . So, I was very happy to have Ron." In time, the Department of Surgery developed a smoother course. Aided by new faculty, competent division chiefs—most of them appointed by Dudrick—and a controlled budget, the UT surgical divisions, in Corriere's words, "ran themselves." These accomplishments formed the nucleus of a new department under the next chair.[7]

In July 1981, Ernst Knobil, an internationally recognized endocrinologist, replaced Tuttle as dean of the medical school. One of Knobil's initial tasks involved the filling of vacancies in several clinical departments, including Otolaryngology, Pathology, and Surgery. "I succeeded in recruiting some outstanding physicians to these positions," Knobil recalled in an interview with Bryant Boutwell for the volume commemorating the school's thirty-year history. Devoting manifold attention to the effort, Knobil had all three of these critical positions filled by the end of his first year. On September 1, 1982, Dr. Frank G. Moody joined the surgical faculty as its chairman, bringing with him eleven years of experience as Chairman of the Department of Surgery at the University of Utah. While Corriere admitted his term as interim chair "was not a lot of fun," he was pleased that the department had earned under his watch a $2 million profit that would smooth the path of his successor.[8]

As mentioned earlier, throughout the first decade of its history, the Department of Surgery established many institutional milestones, while leading the nation into a new era of medical research, education, and patient care. Critical advances in total parenteral nutrition (TPN) revolutionized the treatment of cancer patients. The creation of Hermann Hospital Life Flight, a service unique to the world, paved the way for inventive approaches to trauma care. Moreover, the field of organ transplantation gained remarkable strides in scientific knowledge and clinical expertise. Each outstanding development received energetic approval and support from the departmental chair, Stanley Dudrick.

One of the most significant medical legacies of Stanley Dudrick's tenure as Chair of the Department of Surgery came out of the Division of Immunology and Organ Transplant, headed by Dr. Barry Kahan, which achieved both national and international renown for its groundbreaking role in the development of immunosuppressant drugs and their importance to transplant recipients. In the 1970s, organ transplantation—especially of large organs—was still a fairly new idea. While the procedure had been contemplated since ancient times, it was deemed the stuff of fantasy or science fiction until the mid-twentieth century. The first

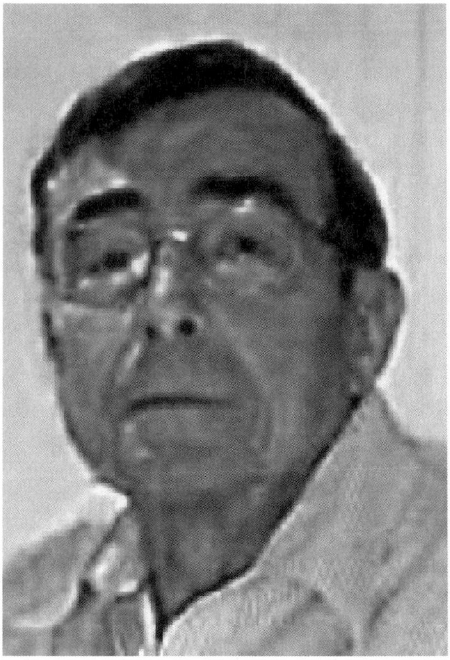

Ronald P. Fischer, MD.

attempt at major organ transplant occurred in 1954, when Dr. Joseph Murray at the Peter Bent Brigham Hospital in Boston conducted the first successful kidney transplantation on a pair of identical twins. With Murray's victory, the age of transplantation had begun.[9]

The Texas transplant era was not far behind. In December 1967, South African cardiac surgeon Dr. Christian Barnard became celebrated around the world for successfully performing the first heart transplant on a human being. On May 3, 1968, Dr. Denton A. Cooley performed the first heart transplant in the United States at St. Luke's Episcopal Hospital in the Texas Medical Center. The patient survived until the following November. On August 31, 1968, just four months after Cooley performed his first heart transplant, Dr. Michael E. DeBakey led a team that performed the first multi-organ transplant, recovering the heart, lungs, and two kidneys from a single heart-beating cadaveric donor and putting the organs into four men. The results were mixed. The lung recipient expired within days, as did one of the kidney recipients. The fate of the other renal transplant patient is unknown. However, the fifty-year-old male heart transplant recipient survived four years—an extraordinary accomplishment so early in the game. On April 4, 1969, Cooley administered the first artificial heart implant on Mr. Haskel Karp, who died of complications four days later, on April 8.[10]

The initial excitement and optimism surrounding the early transplant program quickly faded. Early patients started a good recovery, but then their bodies began to reject the new organs and infection soon developed, most often claiming the patient's life. The high mortality rate hindered the progress of the transplant program. Further, dialysis therapy for end-stage renal disease and the development of heart assistive devices called into question the future use of transplant surgeries. For almost a decade following the first multi-organ surgery in the summer of 1968, DeBakey and colleagues limited their transplant cases to less than sixteen per year. Nevertheless, issues involving transplant patient survival continued to percolate among the medical community. Something was needed to encourage the immune system to preserve the new organs while fighting off infection. X-Ray was an option—but the subsequent dose of radiation often killed the patient. Certain drugs combined with tissue typing produced a higher measure of success. Still, the door remained open for safer, more effective solutions.[11]

Always in search of distinct missions in medical care, Stanley Dudrick embraced the challenge. The development of better immunosuppressive drugs quickly became a goal at the school. This objective acquired considerable speed with the arrival of Dr. Barry D. Kahan to the medical school. As acting head of the transplant program at Northwestern University in Chicago, Kahan possessed a years-long interest with issues regarding immunosuppression and transplant. His quest began in 1960 while engaged in a parallel pursuit of obtaining a doctorate in physiology and a subsequent medical degree from the University of Chicago. Having been awarded the prestigious Danforth Research Fellowship, Kahan received a plum invitation from Aron Moscona, an internationally renowned biologist at the University of Chicago, best known for providing early insight into how cells recognize each other and interact.[12] Moscona needed a research assistant to spearhead his laboratory work, specifically pertaining to issues regarding organ transplantation. Kahan accepted, and as research inevitably goes, ended up following a path of his own. "As time went on," Kahan recalled, "I switched from what Moscona was interested in, which was embryonic tissue transplantation . . . to the question of biochemistry of the transplantation antigens. These are the factors that trigger rejection." Efforts expended in Moscona's lab led to a groundbreaking post-doctoral publication dealing with the isolation of transplantation antigens. An internship at Massachusetts General Hospital and a subsequent career stop at the National Institutes of Health (NIH) eventually put Kahan in the driver's seat of the transplant program at Northwestern. It was here, in 1975, that Kahan became connected with UT-Houston.[13] Stan Dudrick was fascinated by the issues and practices surrounding organ transplant and dreamed of bringing a transplant program to Houston. With preliminary paperwork complete and urologists Joseph Corriere and Bill Connor already on board, Dudrick sent Ted Copeland on a site visit to seek out Kahan at Northwestern. In 1976, Kahan accepted an invitation to come to Houston—with reservations. Like many early faculty, Kahan would be trading a career at a venerable, century-old medical institution with an extensive university hospital system for a brand new school consisting of one building and—most significant to Kahan—no university hospital. Instead, Kahan recalled that the fifty-year-old Hermann Hospital, "had the reputation of being a charity institution."[14]

While Kahan's assumption regarding his future base of operations was correct, Hermann Hospital occupied an important position in the Houston health care community. The hospital was a legacy of Houston entrepreneur-philanthropist George H. Hermann, who upon his death in 1914 willed a sizable portion of his $2.6 million estate toward the building of a public charity hospital. However, as evidenced on opening day in July 1925, the appearance and operations of Hermann Hospital were not that of the average charity hospital. Designed in sixteenth-century Mediterranean style, the five-story structure was flanked by towered, seven-story bays, and had an elegantly tiled entry and lobby. Beautiful wood-paneled hallways and doors led to five operating rooms, a state-of-the-art electric kitchen, and a twenty-ton ice plant. Perhaps best of all, the 100-bed hospital specialized in single-patient rooms—a clear departure from the old-style ward model containing thirty to forty beds per room. "There is no hospital like it in beauty and efficiency in the South," proclaimed the American Construction Association. Many Houstonians agreed, despite the fact that the then–heavily wooded grounds required a fence to keep coyotes and wolves at bay.[15]

Over the succeeding decades Hermann Hospital occupied a central role in Houston's ever-expanding health care mission. By the mid-1970s, the hospital had been home to a thriving nursing school, a pre-natal and child health clinic, a cancer clinic, and a special orthopedic unit for the Arabia Temple Crippled Children's Clinic. The establishment of the Texas Medical Center in Hermann's back yard paved the way for an early arrangement with the Baylor University Medical School. Beginning in 1943, Hermann served as a teaching hospital for the early classes of Baylor students and continued in that capacity until the mid-1950s, when Baylor shifted its alliance to Methodist Hospital. By that time Hermann Hospital had more than doubled in size and capacity, to over 375 beds. Yet the hospital found itself without a medical school.[16] This situation, however, did not last long. As discussed earlier, in 1968, with a clear sense of Hermann's historic and potential role within the Houston medical community, The University of Texas system aligned itself with the hospital. Beginning with the first medical school class in 1971, all UT-Houston students embarked upon regular clinical rotations within "old-style" double doors and "nice colored . . . original" paneling of what was by that time known as "old Hermann." By the end of the decade, on the fourth floor of the hospital, Kahan would begin to create a new organ transplant program.[17]

Years later, a colleague would describe Kahan's first years at UT-Houston as nothing short of a "whirlwind."[18] Within three months his Chicago team of eighteen surgeons, physicians, immunologists, technicians, and social workers had relocated to Houston, setting up shop at Hermann Hospital. Almost overnight, the newly developed Division of Immunology and Organ Transplantation became the largest division of the Department of Surgery. Kahan's momentum was assured by several factors: the fulfillment of funding resources offered by Dudrick during the recruitment process; enthusiastic support from Hermann Hospital Director Bill Smith; and a wide open market for transplants. By the mid-1970s, Baylor surgeons Drs. Michael DeBakey and George Noon had narrowed their transplant specialization to artificial devices. Very few cadaveric or living-related-donor organ transplants were being performed in Houston. For instance, between 1963 and 1976, Baylor never

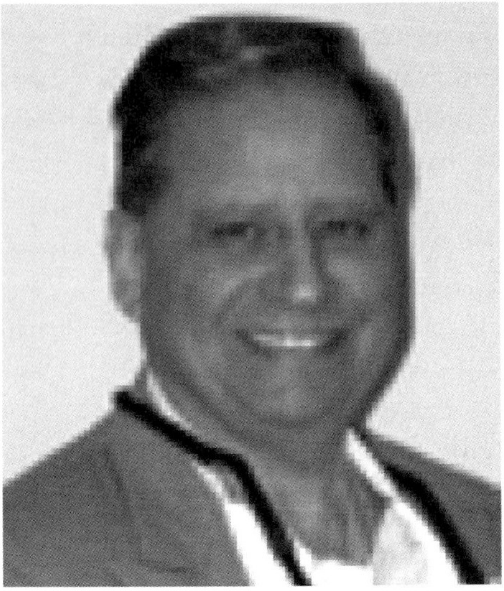

Barry D. Kahan, MD.

exceeded more than sixteen kidney transplant cases per year.[19] Kahan perceived this to his advantage. "I felt pretty comfortable that [Houston] was an environment that no one was really going to compete in," he observed. "In Chicago, we had six programs doing transplants, and one of the problems with that environment is that you have so many people doing something, they become very competitive with each other, and that competition becomes destructive, because if the patient hears from each person how lousy everybody else is, the patient assumes nobody is any good and goes up to Wisconsin. So, I figured that this was a chance to really have an environment in which one did not have that sort of destructive competition."[20]

In the midst of this collegiate atmosphere, during 1977, Kahan welcomed Dr. Charles T. Van Buren, a young surgeon who possessed a bright future within the transplant service. Inspired by a physician father and an early favorite book *Aerosmith,* a 1920s-era classic by Sinclair Lewis about a young doctor's efforts to enter the world of medical research, the arrival of Van Buren to Kahan's division was a destination on an already decades-long dream. Van Buren's potential was already well known to his new superiors. While studying medicine at the University of Pennsylvania in the late 1960s, Van Buren served a three-year stint as research assistant for Stan Dudrick before the latter's departure to Houston. During his residency in Boston, Van Buren met Kahan while on a heart surgery rotation at Massachusetts General Hospital. Having arrived at UT-Houston upon Dudrick's invitation, Van Buren began his term working alongside his former mentor in the Department of General Surgery. However, at Kahan's invitation, Van Buren soon shifted to the transplant service. While his first years would involve considerable on-the-job training, Van Buren felt fortunate to be a first-hand witness to a rapidly changing field. "The thing that was exciting about the transplant service at the time [was] the molecular approach to surgery," Van Buren recalled. In an era where surgery was viewed primarily from an anatomical standpoint, confronting issues regarding transplant patient survival through a molecular lens was intriguingly novel.[21]

After several months of getting organized, putting his team in place, acquiring the requisite licenses, and setting up a transplant center, in May of 1977, Kahan performed the first University of Texas Medical School kidney transplant. By year's end his team would perform the procedure on an additional thirty-one patients. In 1978, the number of renal transplants rose to sixty-three, including a most unusual patient who arrived during the spring. Indian evangelical missionary R. A. C. Paul was living among the Bondos tribe in the remote Indian district of Malkangiri when he became seriously ill. His kidneys failing, the 36-year-old Paul embarked upon a desperate trip across the world to Houston. As he checked into Hermann Hospital, Paul's chances for survival appeared slim. Due to his uncommon blood type, no matching living donor could be found for the young minister. His luck changed when, in early May, Kahan proposed a different route. Instead of waiting for a living donor, Kahan transplanted into Paul the cadaver kidney of a fifteen-year-old girl who had recently died from head injuries in a motorcycle accident. It was a risky venture. "We were concerned about locating a suitable organ for transplant so he could recover and return to India prior to the expiration of his visa," Kahan later explained. However, even though the newly transplanted kidney was not an ideal match, the administration of anti-rejection drugs enabled the donor organ to "function beautifully." Although dependent upon anti-rejection drugs and other precautionary medications for the rest of his life, Paul would not need to lose any of his missionary zeal. In an interview with the *Houston Post*, Kahan predicted Paul's ability to return to the Bondos tribe within a year. In the wake of this triumph with Paul came a groundbreaking collaboration. In 1978, the Medical School's transplant surgeons teamed with heart pioneer Denton Cooley at the Texas Heart Institute to perform at St. Luke's Episcopal Hospital the first heart/kidney transplant.[22]

Meanwhile, research efforts continued, led by Kahan, who focused upon the metabolic characteristics of cyclosporine, which, although toxic, possessed great potential benefit to renal transplant patients. A soil fungus derivative, cyclosporine reduces activity in the immune system by potently blocking the stimulation of T cells while maintaining the activity of B cells, the body's first line of defense.[23] With the aid of cyclosporine, Kahan believed the body would be better able to resist infection--and consequently rejection--of transplanted tissue. Persuaded by conclusions derived in his active UT-Houston laboratory, Kahan proceeded to take the next step. Not only was the use of cyclosporine expected to fight infection, but it might also enhance the progress of transplants—especially kidney transplants—between unrelated, unmatched donors.[24]

However, before the drug could be clinically implemented on a nationwide scale, it needed to be tested. In 1980 the transplant division at UT-Houston was selected, along with the transplant centers at the University of Colorado and University of Minnesota, to conduct a three-phased clinical trial for the federal Food and Drug Administration. All three sites documented that cyclosporine improved graft survival and reduced acute rejection rates. The FDA approved cyclosporine in 1983.[25] The motion opened up a new era in transplant surgery. It was, according to Van Buren, "clearly . . . a quantum jump." Most individuals, he explained, think of medical progress as being a slow, incremental process, but Van Buren mused, "It is more like quantum mechanics . . . with new technology, all of a sudden there will be this jump-shift to a higher level of performance just based on the technology alone. And that clearly was the case from azathioprine to cyclosporine. The success rate before cyclosporine was 35 to 50 percent success. It went up to 80 percent for a one-year success, immediately." The availability of cyclosporine transformed the entire transplant scene. Clinical experimentation now segued into effective clinical practice.[26]

While still in the midst of FDA testing, in 1982, Cooley and Dr. O.

Howard "Bud" Frazier recruited Kahan and Van Buren to assist on a series of cardiac transplants using cyclosporine. By that time, Kahan later admitted, "I was pretty convinced that cyclosporine was going to be useful . . . and [the transplants] were quite successful." The result was that in the midst of the FDA trials, a cyclosporine era formally began in 1982. "In any case, in 1982, when I was pretty convinced that cyclosporine was going to be useful, Dr. Cooley and I embarked on a series of heart transplant patients," said Kahan. "Those were the first hearts that were done in Houston in a number of years." These feats ushered in a groundswell of transplant activity for UT-Houston. By the mid-1980s, Kahan noted, "We were doing 120 kidneys a year. We had about 130 employees in the division, including six PhDs, and a number of technical and support people. It was a very good environment."[27] In less than a decade, the transplant services at Hermann Hospital grew from an initial four-bed unit to occupying half a floor in the old Robertson wing of the hospital to utilizing the entire ninth floor of the newly expanded Jones Pavilion in 1982.[28]

By the mid-1980s, Kahan had masterfully assembled a world-renowned program in transplantation at the Medical School. In addition to organ transplant itself, the program featured innovations in patient care, the training of physicians and researchers, and drug development beyond cyclosporine. One important avenue involved educational outreach. In May 1983, the Medical School hosted the First International Congress on Cyclosporine, which took place in Houston.[29] Over 1,000 delegates attended the sessions, further establishing the Medical School in its role as a pioneer medical center. The purpose of sharing outcomes and effects of cutting-edge research—in this case, cyclosporine—was, quoting Van Buren, to ensure that [the parent institution] becomes "middle of the pack and everybody basically becomes as good as you are . . . That is the challenge always in academics—to constantly be providing new knowledge and then making your previous accomplishments irrelevant as you try to go forward."[30] Between 1954 and 1973, about 10,000 kidney transplants were performed. In 1983, nearly 9,000 transplants were performed in the United States using cyclosporine—with an 85 percent survival rate for the first year.[31]

Investigative studies into newer, potentially less toxic immunosuppressant drugs were another important feature. While the implementation of cyclosporine saved thousands of lives, it was not the last word in transplant. It could be, in fact, lethal. "One of the side effects of cyclosporine that had become pretty obvious in the mid-1980s," reflected Kahan, "was that it was toxic to the kidney." A quest was in order to find drugs that could be used separately or in tandem with cyclosporine. "What we were looking for was synergism," explained Kahan, "because one wanted to reduce the cyclosporine exposure as much as you could."[32] The next effective drug studied was an IL-2 receptor blocker, which is the mainstay of part of the immunosuppression that is used in most transplant patients. The final investigation, explained Van Buren, involved both animal and human studies to research the effects of sirolimus (also known as rapamycin). Over the course of the next ten years, research led by Kahan engaged in tests to reduce the level of cyclosporine, first by 25 or 30 percent, then by 50 percent, then by 80 percent. This led to the division's role in promoting the development of pioneer immunosuppressive lifesavers like cyclosporine (1983), basiliximab (1996) and Rapamycin, or sirolimus (1999).[33]

The UT-Houston Division of Immunology and Organ Transplantation did not stop with procedures involving the kidney. Lessons learned from kidney transplantation initiated groundbreaking work by UT surgeons in the field of liver and pancreatic transplant. After the kidney, the liver was the second organ to be transplanted in humans. Development of a safe and successful procedure took years. Liver physiology, with its complicated nuances, created a long, difficult journey for advocates of surgical transplantation.

Dr. Thomas Starzl, an innovative surgeon at the University of Colorado Medical Center in Denver, pioneered the liver transplant technique in 1963. The patient, a three-year-old child with biliary atresia, did not survive the procedure. Neither did the subjects of four additional transplant attempts. Over the following decade the medical establishment remained pessimistic, as subsequent procedures led by Starzl resulted in high rejection rates. Doggedly optimistic in the face of repeated failure, Starzl continued with his mission. Hopes improved over the following decade as the Colorado team performed numerous transplants, with the term of survival extended to over a year for a quarter to a third of patients undergoing the procedure. However, by 1975, liver transplants by either the Colorado or Cambridge transplant teams produced few long-term survivors. The development of cyclosporine changed the equation. Finally, for Starzl and other surgeons, successful transplantation of the liver—and later the pancreas and lung—was now truly feasible.[34]

In 1985 the Division of Immunology and Organ Transplantation celebrated two major milestones: the first liver and pancreas transplants in Houston. In July, a transplant team headed by Dr. Charles Van Buren, who tutored under Thomas Starzl, conducted at Hermann Hospital the first successful liver transplant in Houston. The recipient was Janice Smith, a forty-seven-year-old woman, who was first diagnosed with biliary cirrhosis, a disease of unknown origin in which the body attacks and destroys its own liver. Upon her initial diagnosis in 1976, Smith was told by one physician to "go home and wait to die."[35] Smith refused. Instead, she fervently searched to learn more about the disease, launched a Houston chapter of the American Liver Foundation—and patiently awaited the arrival of a new liver.

A suitable donor for Smith was finally found in mid-summer 1985, and the groundbreaking surgery was quickly put in motion. However, for the surgeons at Hermann, the operation involved one tense moment after another—beginning with Van Buren's trip to the hospital. The lead surgeon was vacationing in Boston when he received the call regarding a donor for Smith. With just the clothes on his back, Van Buren boarded a People Express flight to Houston. But a thunderstorm delayed his landing in Newark for a connecting flight. With minutes to spare upon landing, Van Buren relayed the urgency to make his connection without sharing the purpose of performing the pending transplant. In a twist of fate hardly recognizable to current readers, Van Buren found assistance in an airline attendant who banged upon on the airplane door until the surgeon was allowed to board. Landing at Hobby Airport, Van Buren drove to Hermann and commenced the operation.[36]

Another surprise was in store. When Van Buren's team opened up Smith to perform the transplant, they discovered unforeseen complications. Smith's hepatic artery was damaged and therefore too "fragile" to be connected to a new liver. In addition, the donor liver had a dual artery supply instead of the usual one line to feed blood into the organ. These

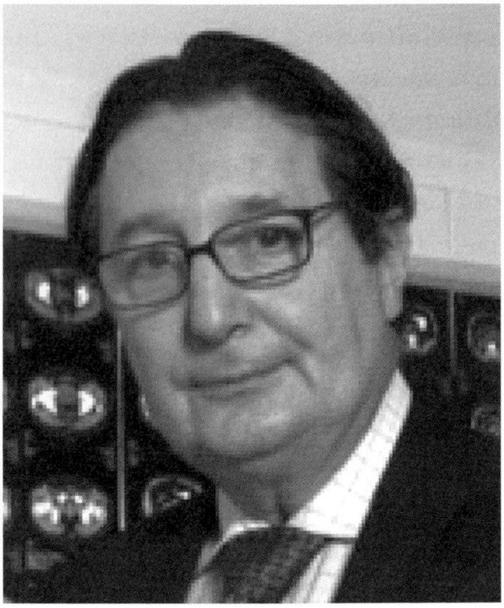

Charles T. Van Buren, MD.

unusual features added extensive risk to the procedure because it forced surgeons to engage in reconstructive surgery for which they had limited time. "We only had four hours from the time [the liver] was removed and the time of transplant," he added. "There was no dialysis equivalent for liver transplant, so you . . . have to do the transplant immediately and the preservation is relatively imperfect."[37] During the reconstruction process, a graft made of pliable material was substituted for Smith's unusable hepatic artery, the main artery leading to the liver. The donor's dual arteries were spliced together and connected to the graft. The surgery lasted a grueling fourteen hours. At the end of it, Van Buren departed for home to catch some needed sleep. But even that plan had complications. He had left his keys in Boston and could not get into his house.[38]

Within a few months, UT surgeons stepped once again into the field of rare gland transplantation when later in 1985, a transplant team led by Kahan performed the first pancreas transplant in Houston. Although the procedure, performed at Hermann Hospital, was certainly a local medical breakthrough, it was still considered quite rare elsewhere—and dangerous. Beginning with the first clinical transplant performed by University of Minnesota surgeons in 1966, the procedure is most often directed toward addressing metabolic disorders associated with Type 1 and Type 2 diabetes, primary pathological contributors to renal failure. It is therefore performed in tandem with or following a kidney transplant. While the initial attempt involved a segmental pancreas graft, the transplantation technique was modified to transplantation of the whole organ by 1973. Rejection, however, was a recurrent event. As of 1984, less than 200 pancreatic transplants had been performed nationwide, with only a 25 percent success rate.[39]

It was Kahan's hope that the experimental transplant performed in Houston could provide a possible remedy for juvenile-onset diabetes. The recipient, a thirty-year-old man suffering a severe case, had undergone a kidney transplant two years earlier. The outset of the operation was promising. Before the procedure, the patient required 200 units of insulin a day to stay alive. That requirement had dwindled down to ten units a few days following the pancreas transferal. With noted achievements within realms of renal, liver, and pancreas transplantation, the UT transplant program further endorsed the UT medical school as a center of academic and clinical excellence. By the close of 1985, UT surgeons had performed over 665 renal and two liver transplants. The positive implementation of the first total pancreas transplantation in Houston spurred a line-up of candidates for the procedure. Following the FDA approval of cyclosporine, surgeons at the Texas Heart Institute invited the UT transplant division to open a satellite transplant service at St. Luke's Episcopal Hospital. An agreement was made, and the first UT facilitated transplants were performed in December of 1986. As the division grew, so did the caseload. "I did six transplants the first year, twelve transplants the next year, and have been doing eighty to 100 transplants a year over the past decade," noted Charles Van Buren. By the late 1990s, the number of renal transplants at Hermann Hospital remained at or above 100 renal transplants per year, while the program at St. Luke's provided over fifty per year.[40]

This impressive output and success fundamentally rested upon the skill and concentration of transplant surgeons on any given day. How was this distinctive focus achieved? In Van Buren's view, compartmentalization was key. "You tend to focus on the task at hand," he said, "because [here is this problem] and this is really annoying. I've got to get that hole closed and that is the way you accomplish what you do . . . There was nobody else to do it. There was work that had to be done and somebody had to do it." At times, the surgeon admitted, the high-pressured responsibility felt overwhelming. "I remember once I was up all night for two nights in a row and I could not make it in clinic—I was just exhausted . . . I got called by the nurse who was on call, yelling at me, saying, "You've got to come here and see these patients!" While the schedule was not very humane, the work within the transplant division during the early decades of transplant at UT-Houston remained very exciting. Van Buren observed, "It was a great place to be: in the fourth-largest city in the United States and one of the more vibrant transplant programs in the country."[41]

While surgical expertise and research perpetuated its growth, the transplant division became even more productive with the establishment of a solid organ donation program. Throughout the first two decades of organ transplant in Houston—from Cooley's first successful human heart transplant in 1968 to Kahan's pancreas transplantation in 1985—the process of organ recovery lacked an organized system. Donors for the major transplant hospitals in Houston—Hermann Hospital, the Methodist Hospital, St. Luke's Episcopal Hospital, and Texas Children's Hospital—were transported from the donor hospital to the transplanting institution. This system of organ transferal worked relatively well for kidney transplant cases, where the patient's life could be sustained through dialysis. However, for other types of organ transplant, including those of the heart and liver, the arrangement was far more precarious. Van Buren recalled, "You have to do the donor and you have to do the transplant immediately." Because no support equivalent to dialysis existed for patients suffering heart or liver failure, surgeons confronted a heated race against time.[42]

In the summer of 1988, transplant surgeons throughout the Texas Medical Center witnessed the beginning of a meaningful organ donor program. It came in the form of "Life Gift" (originally named Gulf Coast Independent Organ Procurement), a nonprofit organization devoted to the procurement of human organs and tissue for transplant. The group was created to recover and preserve organs, to find donors, and to match individuals in need within the Houston area. Life Gift partnered with hospitals to develop an effective, government-regulated donation system to increase the number of donated organs available for transplant.

UT-Houston and Hermann Hospital were among the first to benefit from the affiliation, which has remained fruitful over the decades. In 2010, Memorial Hermann and St. Luke's were two of six Houston-based hospital partners to receive special recognition from the US Department of Health and Human Services for outstanding performance in organ donation and recovery. Over the past twenty-five years, Life Gift has extended service to 109 Texas counties in North, Southeast, and West Texas, and has become in the process one of the most successful organ banks in the country.[43]

Although Stan Dudrick had resigned from the chairmanship in 1980, the department he founded continued to develop many of the pioneering initiatives he originally supported. His participation and influence remained strongly felt throughout the Medical School during the following decade. Dudrick continued to teach as he further advanced the nutritional support and human performance fields. While Dudrick continued a sterling career in teaching and research after resigning the chairmanship, the Department of Surgery effectively moved on as well. A successful interim period led by Dr. Joseph Corriere segued into one of the most outstanding eras in the history of the department. These efforts were fostered by the leadership skills of a newcomer to the medical school, Dr. Frank G. Moody.

CHAPTER 5

The Moody Years, 1982–1994

While growing up in the New England town of Franklin, New Hampshire, it never occurred to Frank G. Moody that he would one day become a world-renowned surgeon. Instead, he dreamed of becoming an architect—an ambition that changed course in due time. He spent his secondary years at Phillips Exeter Academy, graduating in 1946, and joined the military soon thereafter, serving two years as a paratrooper. Upon his release from the service, Moody enrolled at Dartmouth College with the idea of majoring in architecture. However, by this time, his lifelong plan had already begun to fray. While serving overseas, Moody had been assigned to Sapporo, Japan, during the latter part of 1946. To kill time, Moody signed up out of general interest for an evening course in psychology. As it turned out, a preliminary study of psychology evolved into an early introduction to the field of surgery. The professor, as Moody later remembered, was more than a psychologist or a psychiatrist. "He was interested in the biochemistry of schizophrenia, which I thought was fascinating when I was a kid," said Moody.[1] One day, the professor asked Moody if he would like to observe an operation. Moody was thrilled and observed three operations at the Hokkaido University, or what was left of it after being fire-bombed during the war. Viewing the surgeries left a lasting impression on young Moody, who later noted "how interesting that was, and they were so meticulous in what they were doing."[2]

This exposure to the study of medicine put Moody in a different frame of mind. Upon his return to the States, he enrolled at Dartmouth on a pre-med track (1948–1950), continuing his initial graduate work at Dartmouth Medical School (1951–1954). "Initially, I went to [Cornell] with the idea of becoming a psychiatrist," said Moody. "I pursued that with no knowledge of wanting to be a surgeon." His sentiments changed during his final year of medical school when he was assigned as a student psychiatrist at a sanitarium in upstate New York. By the end of his stint there, Moody realized, "I could not spend the rest of my life dealing with [psychological] issues . . . so I went back and talked to the chief of surgery . . . They did not have any matching in those days. The Chief just picked you out, and you would go to work. So, seven years later, I was a surgeon."[3] In 1956, Moody received an MD from the Cornell University Medical College, followed by a residency at the Cornell–New York Hospital Medical Center.

The experiences he gleaned during those seven years at the New York Hospital learning surgery shaped Moody's professional outlook. It was here that he learned the important relationship between clinical surgical practice and scientific training. While he was adept at grand rounds, Moody realized he knew very little about science itself. Therefore, as soon as he finished his residency, Moody took a year off to engage in laboratory work at the Cardiovascular Research Institute at the University of California in San Francisco (UCSF). There, Moody recalled, "I learned the essence of the scientific method. I used to write things down on the back of envelopes, figure it out, get the end result, and do it more formal[ly]. But [in San Francisco], I learned how to systematically approach a problem—develop a question, pose a problem, and stick with it until you solve it."[4] A three-year faculty position at UCSF followed Moody's tenure at the Cardiovascular Research Institute. Armed with both clinical and laboratory expertise, Moody embarked upon a career in academic medicine. After a five-year stint as Director of Digestive Surgery at the University of Alabama, Moody moved to the University of Utah in 1971, where he chaired the Department of Surgery for eleven years.[5]

Surgical treatment of diseases of the digestive system—bariatric surgery for obese patients in particular—became a primary area of interest for Moody. "The obesity surgery turned out to be a God-send in a way," Moody later recalled. "I started in 1975 doing bariatric work, and people used to make fun of me because 'bariatric surgeons work for people who could not do other surgery.' They thought it was disparaging." The process of operating on overtly obese individuals was very difficult and often led to failure. However, Moody saw a need and remained persistent. "I kept going and gradually, [his practice] built and built. Then along comes laparoscopic cholecystectomy—a great contribution to surgery, minimally invasive surgery." Over time, Moody became an expert on the treatment of peptic ulcers, gallstones, inflammation of the intestine, and, increasingly, issues surrounding morbid obesity. By the early 1980s, he had successfully performed over 700 cases.[6]

Administrative officials at UT-Houston took notice. By 1981, the young medical school was entering its second decade. Dr. Roger Bulger was president, and Ernst Knobil, an internationally recognized endocrinologist from the University of Pittsburgh—and first faculty member in the Texas Medical Center to be named to the prestigious National Academy of Science—had been recently appointed dean.[7] Knobil's official charge, he later noted, "was to make this school one of the ten best in the country within a decade."[8] This Knobil was determined to do by developing a strong academic and scientific base on which the clinical initiatives at UT-Houston would rest. Recruitment efforts focused upon research potential. Knobil explained his reasoning: "Most undergraduates couldn't care less about a professor's scholarly contributions. Graduate students, however, are different, and select stars to attach their wagons to. Undergraduate medical students generally respond to people who are good at the bedside and in the classroom, are well-organized, empathetic, and supportive."[9] In addition to being good scientists, each department chair Knobil recruited would possess these characteristics.

An early priority for Knobil centered upon the UT Department of Surgery. Stanley Dudrick had departed during the academic furor the previous summer, and Joseph Corriere was serving as temporary chair. Determined to fill the position in a timely manner, Knobil set his sights on Moody at the University of Utah. One Sunday evening, Moody later recalled, Knobil phoned him and "got right to the point, they wanted me to come down to Houston as the Chair of Surgery, and would not take no for an answer." Content with his research and academic responsibilities out west, Moody quickly refused the offer. Undaunted, Knobil proposed that Moody "at least come to Houston and take a look at the job." Moody continued to hedge. Then, he remembered, "Knobil made me an offer that I could not refuse." The medical school had access to a Lear jet and would fly Moody and his wife, Maja, down to Houston to meet with representatives of the university and Hermann Hospital. The resource potential behind such a bequest captured Moody's attention.

Two days later, a jet carrying Dr. and Mrs. Moody arrived at Hobby Airport. A subsequent tour of the UT medical facilities within the Texas Medical Center left Moody extremely impressed. Houston was a boomtown in the late 1970s and 1980s. Money from the oil and petrochemical industries was flowing into all aspects of community life, not the least of which involved the medical sphere. Bolstered by endowment dollars, the Medical School experienced a huge increase in budget as more and more students enrolled in its various programs. From his post in Salt Lake City, Moody had "watched Stan Dudrick do a wonderful job of getting [the department of surgery] off the ground."[10] By 1981, the school had met its mandate to increase class size to 200 students. Along with class size came a proportional increase in budget.[11]

To Frank Moody, the financial capacity of UT-Houston was startling. The budget quoted by Knobil and Hermann Hospital Director Bill Smith involved "numbers I had never seen before. We weren't talking about thousands of dollars. We were talking about millions of dollars, because they had it in those days." The largesse of the Medical School contrasted sharply with the amounts to which Moody was accustomed. "In terms of my academic program, I was getting $300,000 a year from the State of Utah, because that is about as much as they could scrape up, and the rest, we had to earn, which was okay, but all of a sudden, they were talking about three million dollars a year for the academic program. And they guaranteed that to me for five years . . . So, I said, 'Gee this sounds like an opportunity, I'd better take a look at it.' So, I flew down, and as soon as we landed, I looked around and saw that it was real, things were happening."[12] With a clear view of the immense possibilities UT-Houston had to offer, Moody accepted the chairmanship of the Department of Surgery. According to Dean Knobil, Moody's first day, September 1, 1982, began the "creation of one of the outstanding surgical departments in the country."[13]

Moody came on board with a definite mission: to broaden and strengthen the academic programs in all the surgical divisions. To do so, Moody understood the first task involved taking a thorough inventory of the department. Who did he have on board? What were their academic strengths? How could departmental programs be organized and developed, not only to meet the needs of the medical school but also in

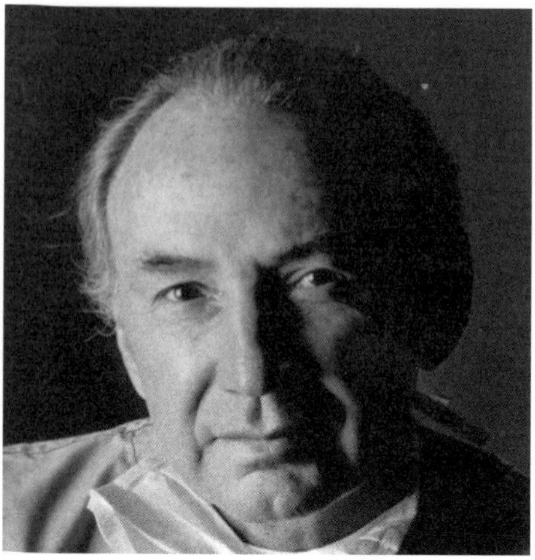

Frank G. Moody, MD, the second chairman of the Department of Surgery.

relation to the larger mission of the burgeoning Health Science Center? While Moody was impressed with many of the faculty, he felt the size of the department itself was too small to create the impact he envisioned. "I wanted to bring in a couple of big hitters," Moody stated later.[14] One area of promise was plastic surgery. Moody recruited Canadian plastic surgeon and burn specialist Donald Parks to head the Division of Plastic Surgery. A graduate of the University of Western Ontario, Parks made the move up Interstate 45 from The University of Texas Medical Branch at Galveston, where he was an Associate Professor of Plastic Surgery and Chief of Pediatric Burn Services at the Shriners Burn Institute.[15]

It was Parks's assignment to develop both the Plastic Surgery Division and a major Burn Center that would work closely with the trauma division at Hermann Hospital. Encompassing all areas of plastic surgery—burns, maxillofacial, microvascular, cleft lip and palate, and reconstructive surgery—the division was a small one during the Moody years. Parks later recalled that it consisted of three full-time faculty, including himself, one resident, and one trainee per year for every two years.[16] Major funding for the fledgling Hermann Burn Center came from the John S. Dunn Foundation, a charitable nonprofit organization dedicated to medical research programs and services in the Houston area—including the first helistop in the Texas Medical Center. While dedicated to trauma care, the Hermann Burn center provided a unique training opportunity for surgical residents to gain experience in burn resuscitation, surgery, and rehabilitation. There was also ample opportunity for residents to gain expertise in minor surgery on both an inpatient and an outpatient basis.[17]

While Parks found the task of developing the Plastic Surgery Division and Burn Center rewarding, the work remained intense. "It is an interesting area, plastic surgery in a major trauma center," Parks admitted, "but it is really hard work, and it never was that easy to recruit individuals to do just major trauma; but we have managed over the years."[18] Parks has remained with the work to the present day. He acknowledges that his proudest achievement is the development of the Burn Center—in conjunction with the John S. Dunn Foundation and what is now the Memorial Hermann Hospital—into a highly respected, comprehensive program.

An early priority for Moody involved the development of Pediatric Surgery at UT-Houston. This endeavor, however, would not be easy. The pediatric surgery program at UT-Houston faced enormous competition from another institution within the Texas Medical Center. Since the mid-1950s, the surgical division at Texas Children's Hospital (TCH) garnered local, national, and international recognition for a wide range of surgical achievements. These included pediatric cardiovascular procedures pioneered by Dr. Denton Cooley, treatment of congenital birth defects, burns and plastic surgery, pediatric anesthesia, and numerous other subspecialties in pediatric surgery.[19] By 1988 more than 2,000 pediatric surgical procedures were being performed at TCH each year by a staff of six general surgeons plus many others in the subspecialty services.[20]

With the lion's share of pediatric initiatives going to Texas Children's Hospital, the UT division of pediatric surgery struggled during its first decade. "There wasn't much pediatric surgery here because of Children's Hospital," Moody remembered. "It takes a lot of chutzpah to think you can compete with Texas Children's. That is one of the biggest things in the world. It is like competing with M. D. Anderson in cancer."[21] Nevertheless, Moody was determined to flesh out the UT pediatric surgery division and put it on the map.

Moody's endeavor began with a search for another division head. Dr. Benjy Brooks, the first to lead the pediatrics division, was still at the helm when Moody arrived. Although the skills and talent that made Brooks a surgical pioneer in Texas remained intact, she was now in her mid-60s and, in Moody's view, limited in her capacity to further build the division.[22] Moody needed a young, dynamic surgeon possessing the capabilities necessary to advance the division.

Moody found it in Dr. Richard Andrassy. Having earned an undergraduate from the Virginia Military Institute and a medical degree from the Medical College of Virginia, Andrassy opted to intern and complete his residency at the Wilford Hall United States Air Force Medical Center in San Antonio. It was here where he first met Frank Moody. In 1972, as Andrassy later recollected, "I was an intern in San Antonio. Dr. Moody came as Visiting Professor, and since I was the low ranking guy on the service, I was his chauffeur to take him back and forth to the visiting officers' quarters."[23] The young intern and senior surgeon from Utah immediately hit it off, continuing a professional relationship over the following decade.

Andrassy was in his second year as Chief of Pediatric Surgery at The University of Texas Health Science Center in San Antonio when Moody approached him in 1984. "Dr. Moody liked the fact that I could do adults as well, since that was what I had been doing all along in the military and in San Antonio, but I was trying mainly to concentrate on pediatric surgery at the time," Andrassy acknowledged. The proposed position was challenging. "The school was only ten years old," noted Andrassy. "A whole lot more senior and more famous surgeons had looked at the job before I got here, and Dr. Moody had really interviewed a lot of good people—it is just that since there was nothing here, most of them did not want to come . . . I was still young enough and maybe stupid enough to say, 'Well, you know, maybe I can make it.'"[24] In the end, Andrassy was offered a potential plum: the position of Chief of Pediatric Surgery at both UT-Houston *and* the M. D. Anderson Cancer Center. Andrassy's task: to build up the pediatric surgery division at each institution. "I was the first pediatric surgeon to work at M. D. Anderson," said Andrassy. "We had to start from scratch, order a bunch of instruments and things. But I had a lot of good help over there. A lot of the older surgeons that had been doing some of the pediatric surgery were very supportive of helping me get started over there."[25]

Andrassy began his mission at UT-Houston in July 1985. Within five years, the UT Division of Pediatric Surgery was in possession of an active clinical and research program. Ongoing projects included the rapid development of a large pediatric surgery service at Hermann Hospital, clinical research on trauma in children, and metabolic aspects of the critically ill pediatric patient. Meanwhile, despite a busy professional travel schedule, Dr. Benjy Brooks continued to teach, engage in clinical research, and promote issues in medical ethics. In 1986, Brooks was awarded the prestigious Horatio Alger award for an outstanding career of accomplishing "great things" through personal initiative and hard work.[26]

That same year, Andrassy initiated a search for a second pediatric surgeon to join the division. After completing a fellowship in Pediatric Surgery at Children's Memorial Hospital in Chicago, Dr. Thomas C. Black joined the team as Assistant Professor of Surgery and Pediatrics. Black's varied research interests inclusive of trauma, immunology, nutrition, and gastrointestinal physiology in neonates fit nicely into the program already initiated by the Division.[27] Numerous papers written by faculty, residents, and students were accepted for publication and presentation at major meetings. In 1989, General Surgery resident Patrick Roughneed's presentation was recognized as the best paper at the Surgical Section of the American Academy of Pediatrics.[28] Frank Moody lauded Andrassy's efforts: "Rich came along and started to add to [the Division] but still low-volume type of stuff, to where now they have eight pediatric surgeons and they are one of the better teaching hospitals in America. They are one of the better teaching services."[29] The expansion and advancement of the Division of Pediatric Surgery under his watch was, Moody later reflected, one of his greatest sources of pride.[30]

The Division of Immunology and Organ Transplantation made tremendous strides during the Moody years. In 1983, the year Moody began his tenure, the immunosuppressive agent cyclosporine received FDA approval. This breakthrough stimulated a wealth of important programs and initiatives under the aegis of Barry Kahan, the director of the Division of Immunology and Organ Transplantation. These included the hosting by UT-Houston of the First International Congress on Cyclosporine in 1983; the opening of a satellite renal transplantation program at St. Luke's Episcopal Hospital in 1986; and the establishment of the instrumental organ donor program, "Life Gift," in 1988.[31] Most important of all were primary developments concerning the organ transplantation process itself. Under Moody's oversight, the new cyclosporine-based regimen encouraged a successful collaboration between Kahan's team and surgeons Denton Cooley and O. H. "Bud" Frazier to reinitiate the heart transplant effort at the Texas Heart Institute. The fruits of this partnership led to further achievements including a successful TMC-based heart and lung transplantation program.[32] Also during these years, UT surgeon Charles Van Buren performed the first liver transplant in Houston in 1985, followed by Kahan implementing the first local pancreatic transplantation procedure in 1986.[33] By the end of the decade the UT organ transplant division was managing one of the largest kidney and liver transplant programs in the country. Transplant efforts were augmented in 1991 with the recruitment of transplant surgeon Dr. Patrick Wood from Creighton University in Nebraska. Over the next five years, Wood led an invaluable Medical Center–wide liver transplant program whereby 157 adult and 110 pediatric liver transplants were performed. While Wood presided over the liver program, Kahan strove to develop a section devoted to pancreatic transplant.[191]

At the heart of these achievements in transplant was a never-ending push by Frank Moody for cutting-edge challenges supported by scientific research. While this stance could ruffle feathers at times, it enjoyed the support of principle academic surgeons within the UT-Houston surgical program. "I was very happy when Moody came," Barry Kahan later recalled in praising Moody's leadership and strong emphasis upon scientific investigation. One important research project involved the relationship between transplant and cancer. "We did a lot of work on cancer," Kahan observed, "because transplantation and cancer are opposite sides of the coin. With transplantation, you want to suppress the immune system, and with cancer therapy, you want to enhance the immune system. So, studying one or the other was very compatible."[35] Another research undertaking involved the field of immunotherapy using antigens to discover what triggered various host responses. According to Kahan, the satisfaction of these and other laboratory discoveries, along with the generous NIH grants to fund them, created "a pretty heady time throughout all that period."[36]

Moody's encouragement and enthusiasm extended to the development of all surgical departments at UT-Houston. However, during the first few years of his leadership, many of the surgical subspecialties, including neurosurgery, orthopedics, and otolaryngology, wanted to form separate, autonomous departments. This quest for independence was not unusual. Indeed, many of the surgical subspecialties in many medical schools throughout the country were following what was during that era a national trend.[37] The petitioning surgeons were "doing a wonderful job. They were excellent people. They were high-quality people," Moody maintained. "But they wanted to develop their presence at the medical school, full time." An important task then involved "trying to overcome political problems and gets these units established and going."[38] Moody encouraged the development and further specialization of each area.

In Moody's view, the nurturing of basic science was essential to quality surgical care. Surgeons needed to understand the pathology behind the procedures performed on the operating table. "I have always felt that if you do not have the surgeon at least trying to do research, you will not be able to get the basic scientists into our world," he observed. The concept of translational research—that of taking a basic problem in the lab, researching it, and transferring the hypothesis to the clinical area—is now a mandated practice in medical schools. However, the idea was very new when Moody first began to explore its possibilities at UT-Houston.[39]

Throughout the 1980s, research conducted by Moody and other UT surgeons grappled with issues behind a popular topic of the era: multiple organ failure after trauma surgery. In earlier years, victims of serious accidents or other physical trauma often expired at the scene. However, improvements in medical transportation and resuscitation techniques ensured that many victims remained alive as they entered the doors of the Hermann Hospital trauma unit. "We would take patients who were terribly banged up," Moody explained, ". . . we made it back to our intensive care units. We made it back to our operating rooms, and we could help them survive . . . Then we began to see this progressive failure of organs about four to five weeks after we patched them up."[40] "We just asked the question of why these people seemed to make it initially but then die."[41] Moody's extensive research effort in gastroenterology steered him to some possible conclusions. "Our thought was . . . that it has something to do with the gut . . . because the bacteria we would find in these people were from the guts."[42] The issue, Moody believed, provided UT surgeons an opportunity to develop a research grant in trauma surgery.

To fully study the question, Moody and fellow UT surgeons Thomas Miller and Stuart Myers spearheaded a full-scale research endeavor. In 1988, Moody initiated a research grant entitled, "Pathogenesis of Multiple Organ Failure."[43] This led to the Trauma Research Center to be implemented at Hermann Hospital. Funded by the National Institutes of Health (NIH), the Trauma Research Center began as a five-year research project to integrate basic science into research activities regarding trauma care.[44] Moody insisted that a certain percentage of the surgery faculty be devoted to research. "I brought people in who had the capacity to do meaningful research," Moody explained. "I would spike them $100,000 or so each year for the first three years . . . to get their labs going."[45] During the first year, new methods of research, computer facilities, and a microbiology laboratory were integrated into the project.[46]

The beauty of the endeavor lay in its multidisciplinary format. The Trauma Research Center at Hermann Hospital occupied the same research space as practicing doctors in the basic sciences. It became then, a source of opportunity for surgeons to work in the laboratory with investigators from other fields. "It not only had surgeons but it also had physiologists involved," noted Moody, "and that fit in very nicely with the school's [mission]"as envisioned by the first medical school dean, Cheves Smythe.[47] "We actually made that work very well," said Moody. "It was a good relationship with Physiology especially, and what it meant for me as a chairman was that I could assign young surgeons to work with some of the basic scientists in learning about the techniques they used . . . we had a transition from basic bench research to the trauma unit, the clinical trauma patients."[48] The bridge created by the Center between the basic sciences and clinical practice marked a notable achievement during Moody's tenure as chair. "We were very successful in academic output, and the residents decided to get very interested in working in the lab, which is what I worked on to try to entice them to come in for a couple of years and enjoy the fruits of their labor."[49] While changes in health care delivery and abbreviated length of hospitalization decreased the patient load at Hermann from 800 beds in 1982 to 450 beds ten years later, the UT-Houston surgical training program remained unaffected.[50]

Importantly, out of the collaboration came vast improvement in intensive care protocols—so much so that instances of multiple organ failure have become increasingly rare. Today, Moody observed, "we are so good at treating the underlying physiology, pathophysiology that basically they wiped out the disease . . . people are still dying of multiple organ failure, but they do not die as often as they used to because of the good care that they are getting in the intensive care units . . . We were very early in what they are now calling translational research . . . So, it has been fun to be part of that history."[51] The laboratory achievements produced by UT surgeons and scientists not only guaranteed fifteen years of additional NIH funding, they enabled the Department of Surgery to gain widespread national recognition. "It was very exciting," Moody recalled. "We began to be known out there as being something other than just a training program for people to practice in Texas."[52] As a result, Moody explained, increasing numbers of "quality" medical school and residency candidates began to seriously eye the department's potential as an effective launch pad for their medical careers.

Throughout the ten-plus years of his leadership, Moody continually searched for new challenges and opportunities to stimulate the education of students and residents. Although only 10 to15 percent of medical students choose surgery as a career, Moody strove to instill within this group the best medical academia had to offer. For instance, he was the first to implement the practice of problem-based learning at The University of Texas Medical School.[53] In Moody's view, this shift in the general education process, from formal lectures to small-group problem-solving sessions, helped ensure a deep appreciation and understanding of the surgical sciences. "It was fun," Moody observed, "to have an idea, take it to the laboratory, then it works or it does not work. If it does not work, you go at it from a different angle and eventually get it to work."[54] Moody also believed problem-based learning was vital to discovering effective means of navigating the multiple challenges inherent in the health care system of the 1980s. Surgical residents, skilled in the clinical arts, were also encouraged to become surgical scientists by spending considerable time in the laboratory. One such individual was Dr. Rafik Ghobrial, who completed a PhD in immunology during his surgical residency, and actively worked on the Trauma Research grant and a Digestive Disease training grant also established with NIH funding in 1988.[55] The emphasis Moody placed upon the blending of clinical practice with laboratory science, upheld by his successor, Richard Andrassy, remains a strong UT tradition today. While Moody emphasized the importance of academic research, he worked tirelessly to strengthen the clinical side of medical education as well. It did not take Moody long to engage with this aspect. By the time of Moody's appointment as UT Chair of Surgery, the medical school was suffering a dearth of charity patients used for clinical teaching. Competition from the more modernized facilities in the Texas Medical Center, in particular St. Luke's Episcopal Hospital and the Methodist Hospital, compelled Hermann Hospital to shrink its patient caseload. This was an alarming development for UT-Houston. Dr. John C. Ribble, the Dean of the Medical School from 1986 to 1994, recalled the situation. "We were being reviewed by the Liaison Committee on Medical Education (LCME), and we were being told that we were marginal in the number of patients that we had available for our educational program . . . We were doing hand flips to show we had adequate numbers of patients."[56] The consequences of the Hermann downsizing became immediately apparent to Moody. "When I first came here, the first letter on my desk was the fact that they were going to put us on probation. That is serious because if you are on probation, you cannot recruit residents."[57] He also understood the importance of buying time. A new general hospital was in the making that would drastically change the current circumstances. Moody later credited Dr. John Potts for helping to resolve the crisis: "He joined us within a few months, and had the program off probation in six months. The program has received unconditional approval ever since, and is stronger now than at any other time in its history."[58]

In 1986 the Harris County Hospital District (HCHD) began construction on a new facility in northeast Houston: the Lyndon Baines Johnson General Hospital (LBJ). The Hospital District, approved by Harris County voters in November 1965, was established to provide medical care for all residents throughout the county. Shortly after its creation, the HCHD took control over the two existing city-county health care institutions, Ben Taub Hospital and Jefferson Davis Hospital. Twenty years later, issues of age and lack of modernization compelled the HCHD to address the future of their flagship institutions. In 1986, a new 578-bed

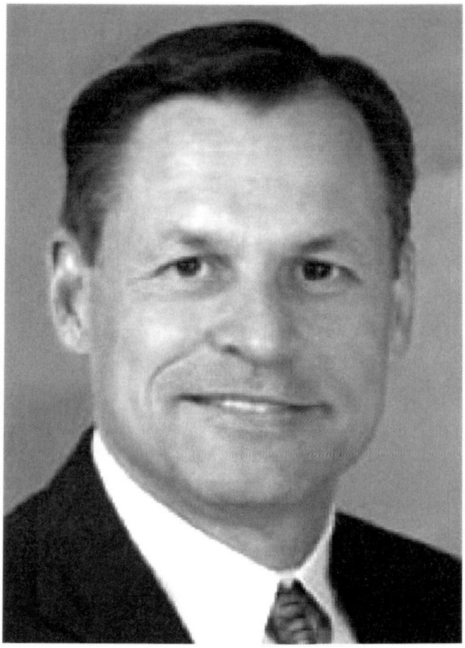

John Potts, MD.

Ben Taub General Hospital, the primary teaching hospital for the Baylor College of Medicine, supplanted the original building next door. And, three years later, the HCHD opted to close the old Jefferson Davis Hospital in favor of the freshly constructed, 328-bed LBJ Hospital. Shortly after the opening of LBJ Hospital in 1989, the Harris County Hospital District joined UT-Houston in approving an affiliation agreement that enabled the school to provide medical staff for LBJ and five of the District's neighborhood health centers.[59]

The partnership proved a boon to the educational initiatives at UT-Houston. "With the addition of LBJ," former Dean Ribble observed, "we had more patients than we knew what to do with, along with an abundance of student training opportunities."[60] Moody was pleased as well. While Hermann kept a good share of low-resource patients, Moody noted that "LBJ became so overloaded . . . that they were very happy for us to offload a lot of cases. So, we filled up very quickly."[61] The UT clinical educational program was back and running "at a good pace," with plenty of money created for resident slots. As a result, the surgical resident program grew substantially in trauma, pediatrics, and other clinical-related fields.[62] Today LBJ Hospital continues to play a fundamental role within the UT Department of Surgery in terms of patient care, research, and the training of young surgeons and faculty.[63] Indeed, the affiliation with LBJ Hospital is viewed by some of the surgical faculty as one of the milestones in the history of the department. "LBJ has been the most rewarding thing for the residency program," said Eduardo Souchon. "They get a great experience, and the cases here, I would say, are more complicated than the cases that you see at Hermann as far as elective surgery is concerned. The elective cases here are the most complex—big tumors, big hernias, big everything." Souchon noted that many of the hospital's patients tend to put off medical care until the problem can no longer be ignored. But this provides the residents with opportunities they might not see in most other hospitals. All of this, in Souchon's view, makes LBJ one of the best teaching institutions in the state.[64]

By summer 1994, Frank Moody felt it was time for him to step down as department chair and turn those responsibilities over to someone new. As he did so, Moody bequeathed a lasting legacy. During his chairmanship, Moody's profound enthusiasm for education, research, and clinical practice proved an unending source of stimulation and encouragement for students, residents, and faculty. His ideas regarding trauma research, the pathogenesis of multiple organ failure, the development of surgical science in space, and many other initiatives kindled among his fellow surgeons a never-ending quest for new knowledge and experiences. An outstanding teacher, Moody inspired the development of problem-based learning methods within the various divisions. Overall, Moody's tenure as chairman created a solid academic department nationally recognized for exceptional achievements in academic research, clinical practice, and surgical education.[65]

On August 15, 1994, the Medical School's dean, John Ribble, asked Dr. Richard J. Andrassy, head of Pediatric Surgery at the medical school, to take over as interim chair. After a nine-month search and interviews with several candidates, the committee recommended that Andrassy be appointed permanently as Chair of the Department of Surgery. "I was very happy just being Chief of Pediatric Surgery and a busy clinician," said Andrassy, years later. "But I had learned a lot about managed care during that period of time, trying to build up referrals for pediatric surgery here. So, since I understood the business side of medicine, Dr. Ribble then asked me to take the permanent job, which I did in 1995." Frank Moody could not have been more pleased with his successor. Ten years earlier, he had personally recruited Andrassy to develop what became a clinical and nationally recognized program in pediatric surgery. Now Moody was passing the baton with a confident eye towards the future.[66]

CHAPTER 6

The Andrassy Era and a Maturing Department

"I do not come from a medical family, but as far back as I remember … I always wanted to be a doctor." —Richard J. Andrassy

Richard John Andrassy formally took over as Chair of the Department of Surgery in the spring of 1995, after serving for nine months on an interim basis. Although he never aspired to a department chairmanship, he was uniquely suited for this responsibility. Even in his youth, he had wanted to be a medical doctor. He was born on August 15, 1946, in Perth Amboy, New Jersey, to Jay William and Laurabelle (Gillen) Andrassy. The family soon moved to New Providence, a small New Jersey town located along the Passaic River, a bucolic community that seemed far removed from the urbane metropolis of New York City, just twenty-two miles to the east. Youthful pastimes were simple: "I spent most of my time either ice-skating, playing hockey on the river, or floating down on a raft, shooting squirrels and things like that," Andrassy remembered.[1] Baseball was a particular pleasure, spurred by the opportunity to play on the New Jersey Little League All-Star team when he was just seven years old. The young Andrassy possessed a thoughtful side as well. Around the same time he was playing for the New Jersey All-Stars, he became closely acquainted with the family doctor who lived down the street from him; an association that opened the door to the fascinating world of medicine.[2]

Although his interest deepened in high school, boyhood temptations kept Andrassy academically off-kilter during his early years. "I was not a very good student before tenth grade," he admitted. "But I figured that if I really wanted to be a doctor, I'd better get on the stick."[3] As a student at New Providence High School, Andrassy began to take a serious interest in studying. He became an avid reader, especially of history, and subsequently his grades improved. "It was a big change in my life," Andrassy noted, but being an ardent athlete, "I did not even want to tell the other guys that I was a really good student."[4] It was the first of several times in Andrassy's life where he grasped an opportunity to reinvent himself.

A part-time job introduced Andrassy to a possible future as a surgeon. During his senior year of high school, he worked at the Muhlenberg Hospital in nearby Plainfield, New Jersey. "I got a job, first shaving patients in the operating room and then assisting and being a scrub tech," he remembered. "I also was the janitor in the OR on the weekends."[5] His assigned tasks provided many opportunities to watch surgeons in action. Especially appealing to Andrassy was the essential speed, concentration, and intensity the practice of surgery required. At one point, Andrassy became a patient himself. "I was ready to go out of town for the weekend with a bunch of guys, and had belly pain," he recalled. A consequent emergency appendectomy sealed his interest in the field of surgery.[6]

By the end of his senior year, Richard Andrassy appeared well-appointed for the next phase of his life. In addition to a stimulating part-time job, Andrassy stood at the top of his class, serving as both senior class president and captain of the baseball team. These credentials paved the path to a promising future after graduation. But which direction should the young Andrassy take? Military school had the greatest pull, since military service occupied an important place within the Andrassy family heritage. Andrassy's father, a former marine stationed in the Pacific during World War II, survived the brutal battles at Guadalcanal and Bougainville as well as an explosion that ripped his ship apart upon its return to the United States. "My father always wanted me to go to military school," Andrassy recalled, "and I had always watched the TV programs about West Point."[7] During the spring of 1964, he received appointment offers from the United States Military Academy at West Point and the United States Air Force Academy, but he eventually selected another: the Virginia Military Institute (VMI). In addition to a superior military education, the school offered Andrassy both a full-fledged sports scholarship and an introductory path to a medical career.

The baseball team at VMI was in need of some good recruits, particularly a pitcher, and school recruiters believed Andrassy fit the bill.

Although he played catcher in high school, Andrassy had developed a really good fastball over the years. "I wound up actually pitching a lot, even though my scholarship was for catching," he recalled. Playing for a small school like VMI made for an exciting experience as Andrassy played catcher, pitcher, or sometimes first base, often at times to his physical detriment. "You get so beat up as a catcher. In those days, they would throw the bat, they would try to run you over, and some of those guys were big. I was 160 pounds in college and these 220s would try to run you over and knock you out . . . I broke my nose, my fingers, and have a knee replacement." Nevertheless, he noted, "It was fun."[8]

Exciting as a sports scholarship was to Richard Andrassy, VMI also provided a solid chance to get into medical school. As a freshman in the fall of 1964, Andrassy looked forward to studying under one of the most notable—and colorful—faculty members in the history of the institute. For forty years, beginning in 1928, Robert P. "Doc" Carroll, a one-armed, tobacco-chewing professor imparted his wisdom to countless biology majors at VMI and was instrumental in placing many of them in medical and dental school. "You could hardly understand him because he was chewing tobacco and spitting while he was writing on the blackboard," Andrassy reminisced. But, "if you did well, you got into medical school easily."[9] There was also another incentive. The United States was engaged in a full-fledged war in Southeast Asia. "If you flunked out or got kicked out, they immediately sent you to Vietnam in those days," said Andrassy.[10]

Determined to succeed at VMI, Andrassy tackled the rigorous curriculum and an inflexible sports schedule. Dating and other outside activities were exceedingly rare for him. "You could only go out until 12 o'clock on Saturday night anyway," Andrassy later explained, "so I just stayed and played sports and studied."[11] Sticking to campus paid off for Andrassy, and he excelled academically at VMI. He began to look at medical schools but being short on time and money, interviewed at only three schools: Bowman Gray School of Medicine, the University of Virginia School of Medicine and the Medical College of Virginia (MCV). "I did it all in one trip, basically," Andrassy recalled. "By the time I got back to VMI, I had an acceptance to the Medical College of Virginia."[12] Andrassy quickly accepted and began looking forward to arriving in Richmond the following year with several classmates from VMI.

It was only later in life that Andrassy had time to reflect upon the historical uniqueness of his undergraduate experience at VMI. The Virginia Military Institute is steeped in Civil War history. Early cadets attending VMI had a future Confederate general, Thomas Jonathan "Stonewall" Jackson, as a professor of philosophy and artillery. In addition, cadets from the school were to play an instrumental role in the Battle of New Market, Virginia, one of the most studied small battles of the Civil War. On May 15, 1864, two hundred and fifty VMI cadets were called out in an effort to halt part of a multi-pronged Union advance up the Shenandoah Valley. The youngest participating cadet was fifteen, the oldest twenty-one. The steadiness and audacity displayed by the cadets under heavy fire at New Market eventually broke the Union line.[13] Years later, the historical contributions of VMI and former professors pervaded the culture of the school. "There is a big statue of Stonewall Jackson as you come out of the barracks," reminisced Andrassy. Moreover, "The Cadets of VMI are the only ones that fought in a real war, so it is the only military school in the country where the capes are red underneath."[14] While his rigorous study schedule gave Andrassy little time to appreciate it as a student, the unique environment of VMI stimulated a life-long interest in Civil War history.[15]

In the spring of 1968, a different conflict threatened to upset Andrassy's long-awaited plans for medical school. The American war in Vietnam had reached a crescendo, with over 540,000 troops on the ground in Southeast Asia, and the military desperately needed fighter pilots. As one of the only six in his class at VMI to earn the 1P flight classification, Andrassy was immediately commissioned for flight school. Luckily, fortune was on his side. Andrassy's plight captured the notice of Gen. James W. Humphreys, MD, a graduate of both VMI and MCV and Surgeon General of the United States Air Force. Humphreys took a helicopter down to VMI, landed on the parade ground, and treated the young cadet to a fried chicken dinner. At the end of the visit, Humphreys told Andrassy: "You are a really good student . . . and you can help the air force and the country better if we trained you and let you be a doctor and not be a pilot right now."[16] Humphreys pulled some strings, and a few weeks later, Andrassy possessed a military deferral that enabled him to remain on active duty, yet go directly to medical school on a full scholarship. Andrassy entered the MCV as a second lieutenant. By his third year, he had achieved the rank of captain.[17]

As Richard Andrassy progressed through medical school, his interests evolved. While he briefly considered a career in child psychiatry, surgery—orthopedic surgery in particular—continued to have the greatest appeal. "I was thinking along the lines of pediatric sports medicine," Andrassy remembered. Then another avenue presented itself: pediatric oncology. As a third-year student in pediatrics, Andrassy had the good fortune to work under renowned pediatric oncologists including Dr. Hal Mauer, who later instigated the noted Intergroup Rhabdomyosarcoma Study, and Dr. Walter Lawrence, a future president of the American Cancer Society. In his fourth year, Andrassy rotated onto the pediatric surgery service. The chair of the pediatric surgery division, Dr. Arnold M. Salzberg, left a lasting impression on the young intern. "Dr. Salzberg was just fascinating to me . . . He did all kinds of surgery. He seemed to be the master surgeon to me, with a great attitude, but really down-to-earth." Andrassy fondly recalled that Salzberg would take his students out for a cigar and a little Scotch. He was very nice to the students and residents, but could be quite strict as well and was known to send those who failed to meet his standards to stand in the corner. One particular encounter was especially memorable: when an unfortunate resident was sent to the corner, Salzburg invited Andrassy to fill in and help with the case. Under Salzberg's influence, Andrassy thus began to seriously contemplate a career in pediatric surgery.[18]

Another important individual for Andrassy at MCV was the famous surgeon and researcher, Dr. David Hume. A member of the team that performed the first successful kidney transplantation at the Peter Bent Brigham Hospital in Boston, Hume was a pioneer in endocrine and vascular surgery as well as neuroendocrinology research. In 1956, he became the Stuart McGuire Professor of Surgery and Chairman of Surgery at MCV. Described as a "restless genius" and "superb teacher," Hume instilled in many of his students a profound spirit of inquisitiveness and joy of discovery.[19]

Under Hume, the most promising students received special attention, but in Andrassy's case, this proved to be a mixed bag. "I worked for him in his lab, which allowed me to get paid to study. But I also did a lot of chores for him. On Saturday mornings I would meet him early in the morning at the Skull and Bones across the street from MCV. He would give me a list of chores for the day, which would include getting his car washed, picking up his laundry, going to the liquor store, and other issues that I would do before I got to go to the lab."[20] Despite his abuse of Andrassy's time, Hume also knew promise when he saw it. Impressed with Andrassy's intellect and performance in his laboratory, Hume invited the young medical student to remain at MCV for his internship and residency training in general surgery.[21]

The United States Air Force thought otherwise, however, and Andrassy still had a military commitment. Upon his graduation from MCV in 1972, he received orders to report to Lackland Air Force Base in San Antonio, where a surgical internship awaited at the Wilford Hall USAF Medical Center. During that era, Andrassy later explained, the organization of internships resembled a pyramid model. "There were twenty-two new interns at Wilford Hall. They were going to move to twelve and then six and then down to four by the time we finished." Andrassy did not possess one of the original slots. "I was only going as a preliminary intern with the idea that I would be there for one year. Then I would go back and train at MCV in general surgery with the hopes of getting into pediatric surgery."[22] However, in May of 1973, Andrassy learned of Hume's untimely death in a plane crash. His plans for a full residency at MCV were dashed, filling him with uncertainty. In those days, Andrassy later noted, there were no match programs or written guarantees, and his plans to return to MCV were based on a handshake and an oral commitment. He found himself in the uncertain situation of having no residency agreement. Fortunately, several senior residents pleaded Andrassy's case to the Wilford Hall faculty and convinced them to keep him for the second year. A third year followed, and by then, said Andrassy, "I just went straight on through" as one of four residents who finished the five-year program. During this time, Wilford Hall was an extremely busy place, and the years in San Antonio comprised some of the most important of Andrassy's life. [23]

During the late 1960s and early 1970s, the Wilford Hall USAF Medical Center was an exceptional place to do a residency. With 1,100 beds, it was the largest and busiest US Air Force hospital in the world. Due to the extraordinary caseload created by the war in Vietnam, the daily schedule for elective surgeries extended from 7:00 in the morning until 11:00 at night. "We were on every other night in the hospital and on backup call by beeper on our nights off," Andrassy recalled. "Most of the time we might get home for four, five hours." Although very hectic, the large caseload provided excellent training for residents. "By our second year," Andrassy remembered, "we were doing all kinds of vascular and large [hernia] cases and endocrine cases—just with the junior resident."[24] However, Wilford Hall did not have a rotation in pediatric surgery. In order to train further in the specialty, Andrassy received permission to spend his second year of residency at the Santa Rosa Children's Hospital in San Antonio.

Pediatric surgery in particular fascinated him, especially pertaining to childhood cancer. Pediatric surgery was relatively new on the scene when Andrassy selected it as his specialty of choice, and pediatric oncology even more so. Modern pediatric surgery was born from the efforts of Dr. William E. Ladd, acknowledged today as the "father" of pediatric surgery.[25] Working out of Boston Children's Hospital (BCH) in the early 1920s, Ladd became distressed by the quality of surgical care offered to infants and small children. General surgeons traditionally discounted the physiological distinction between children and adults. A Boston surgeon once expressed to Ladd, "Anyone who could operate on a bunny rabbit could operate on newborns." Determined to prove otherwise, Ladd intensely studied the various surgical problems of infants and children and meticulously examined the results of their treatment.

Utilizing a wealth of new information, Ladd developed over the years new procedures and methods of pediatric care. His work addressed the correction of various congenital defects, including intestinal malformations, and he became the first surgeon to save a child with esophageal atresia. At BCH, Ladd developed the first training program for pediatric surgeons. In 1938, Ladd's Boston protégé, Dr. Robert E. Gross, made history when he performed the first surgery to correct a congenital heart defect. His patient, seven-year-old Lorraine Sweeney, suffered from a patent ductus ateriosus, a malady consisting of a persistent abnormal opening between the pulmonary artery and the aorta, a condition that in the 1930s was considered a death sentence.[26]

In the ensuing years Gross and Ladd collaborated to write the first modern American textbook on child surgery, the 1,000-page *Abdominal Surgery of Infancy and Childhood,* published in 1941. Through extensive analysis and procedural detail, the manual emphasized that children should not be treated as miniature adults. Their needs are different, the authors noted, and the best care for children is given by surgeons who make pediatrics their life's work.[27] With this concept in mind, Ladd recommended to the newly organized American Board of Surgery (ABS) that an avenue be developed to certify surgeons with a special interest in children.

Despite several impressive surgical milestones, the field of pediatric surgery grew slowly. Traditional surgeons hesitated to give it a respected place at the table. For instance, Ladd's proposal to the American Board of Surgeons for pediatric certification took over thirty-three years to come to fruition. "It was not until 1976 that pediatric surgery achieved recognition as a separate specialty," Andrassy remembered. "Even in 1977, the year I finished my residency, there were few boarded pediatric surgeons."[28]

Newer still was Andrassy's chosen subspecialty, pediatric surgical oncology. It formally began in 1948, when observations by Dr. Sidney Farber, later known as the "father" of modern pediatric pathology, demonstrated the benefits of chemotherapy for treating childhood acute lymphoblastic leukemia.[29] Farber's discovery encouraged further development of treatments, preventatives, and cures for childhood cancer. Reflecting upon the measured progress in childhood cancer research over the next two decades, Andrassy noted, "I got interested in pediatric surgery and cancer in children, because a lot of kids were dying back in the late 1960s which now there are treatments for."[30] Upon completion of his residency in 1977, Andrassy trained three additional years at the University of Southern California and the Los Angeles Children's Hospital, where he completed fellowships in Pediatric Surgery and Pediatric Surgical Oncology.[31] During that time, Andrassy continued with his developing interest in enteral nutrition. He collaborated on studies involving early enteral, tube, and jejunostomy feeding.[32] By the end of his term in California, Andrassy possessed an exceptional résumé. In 1980, he belonged to a very small circle of pediatric surgeons in the United States thoroughly trained in adult general surgery, pediatric surgery, and pediatric cancer surgery.

Andrassy's expertise in all three arenas profoundly influenced his career in the coming years. Indeed, the consequences were almost immediate. "I was too well-trained for [the air force] to send me into combat or send me overseas," Andrassy later observed.[33] Instead, he opted to return to Wilford Hall Medical Center, where he could make use of his skills as a pediatric surgeon. But along came an interesting twist of fate. Andrassy's stellar academic and clinical reputation was not the only aspect appreciated by his superiors. Some took notice of his athletic ability. Dr. Larry Fontenelle, the powerful Chief of Surgery at Keesler Air Force Base in Biloxi, Mississippi, was drawn to Andrassy's experience playing high school and college baseball. The Department of Surgery had an amateur team. Each year the surgeons played their heated rival, the Department of Internal Medicine, and each year the surgeons lost.[34]

Weary of the annual drubbing, Fontenelle took matters into his own hands. He personally assembled a winning team by adding athletic talent to the list of valued qualifications for departmental recruits. Several young surgeons had played university baseball and one had played for West Point. Once he learned of Andrassy's baseball experience, Fontenelle pulled a few strings. Shortly thereafter Andrassy received a transfer from Lackland Air Force Base to Keesler. The following spring, the surgeons had built a formidable team. "It was totally unfair, in fact," Andrassy recalled. "We had a big pep rally the night before the game," and "we killed them, 17 to 1!"[35] The same scenario continued for at least three more years.

Fontenelle's aspirations for Andrassy extended far beyond a worthy addition to the departmental baseball team. He wanted a highly qualified pediatric surgeon, especially one that did a lot of general surgery as well. Andrassy remembered, "He brought me in and said, 'This is a great opportunity for you. You can be the chief of general surgery and pediatric surgery and program director, and in a couple of years when I step down, you can be Chairman of Surgery.'"[36] Andrassy accepted, joined the Department of Surgery, and quickly rose from the status of fellow to Chief of General and Pediatric Surgery.

In July 1980, Andrassy welcomed his first intern. Dr. Kevin Lally, a graduate of the US Air Force Academy in Colorado Springs, and Tulane University Medical School, arrived at Keesler intent upon a career in academic surgery. "The faculty [at Keesler] was more academically focused than most, and that was my strong interest," Lally later explained.[37] However, through working with Andrassy, Lally professed, "I got very interested in pediatric surgery." Since military hospitals were not structured to allow time for outside research, Andrassy arranged for Lally to obtain his first research fellowship at Boston Children's Hospital.[38] While there, Lally completed a two-month rotation in pediatric surgery, and, in the process, met his future wife, Pam Fisher, the rotating pediatric resident. The fortunate results of Andrassy's mentorship with Lally sparked an enduring and fruitful colleagueship. Within a few short years, Lally would join Andrassy on the faculty at UT-Houston and eventually succeed his mentor as Chief of Pediatric Surgery.

In 1983, The University of Texas at San Antonio beckoned Andrassy back to Texas. He joined the faculty as Associate Professor of Surgery and Pediatrics and was soon promoted to Chief of Pediatric Surgery. Two years later, at the wooing of Dr. Frank Moody, Andrassy moved to Houston. Moody needed a division chief of pediatric surgery. At the same time, Dr. Charles Balch, the new chief of surgery at M. D. Anderson, was in search of an experienced pediatric surgeon to join his staff. "They were initially looking for somebody a lot more senior," Andrassy remembered, "a previous chief of a big children's hospital."[39] However, with no real pediatric department in place at UT-Houston, very few senior academic surgeons were interested in finishing their careers in such fledging circumstances. Andrassy represented an enticing alternative. He was young, highly motivated, and uniquely qualified for both positions. "I was one of the few in the country that had training in cancer surgery as well as pediatric surgery," Andrassy explained. "So [Moody and Balch] made this new position where I would be the Chief at both places." In July 1985 Andrassy assumed a joint appointment as Chief of Pediatric Surgery at UT-Houston and Chief of Pediatric Surgery at M. D. Anderson. It was an exceptional opportunity, and as he noted later, "There were only a couple of places in the country that you could go and be a pediatric surgeon that mainly did cancer."[40] In assuming this position, Richard Andrassy not only became the premiere head of pediatric surgery at

M. D. Anderson, but the first academic pediatric surgeon to practice in Houston.

For several decades, pediatric surgery had thrived within the private practice sector, yet remained virtually nonexistent inside Houston's academic medical institutions. In 1946, Dr. Luke W. Able, graduate of The University of Texas Medical Branch at Galveston, was the first pediatric surgeon to set up practice in Houston.[41] When he arrived, the Bayou City was undergoing enormous change. The oil and petrochemical industries, firmly established during the war years, continued to transform Houston and surrounding Harris County. Downtown development flourished as construction extended along Main, Fannin, Travis, Milam, and Louisiana streets. A new array of contemporary office buildings altered the city skyline.[42]

Central to Houston's growth were the effects of the postwar baby boom. Fathers, sons, and sweethearts were coming home, entering the workforce, buying homes, and starting families. Between 1940 and 1950, the population in Houston increased by 54 percent, a boom that persisted into the 1960s.[43] The extraordinary surge in Houston's child population increasingly called for specialized pediatric services. Determined to effectively contribute to this need, Able delayed the launching of his practice and briefly left Houston to train under pediatric surgeons Ladd and Gross at Boston Children's Hospital.[44] He returned to Houston in 1948.

In the late 1940s, fewer than twenty pediatricians practiced in Houston, and no children's hospital of any kind had been established. This fact forced Able to not only operate in adult hospitals, but provide around-the-clock care as well. "It kept me running," he later remembered. "Before surgery, if you couldn't start the IV, you couldn't do the case. In those days, there wasn't a recovery room. You recovered your own patients. The joke around town was, I not only operate on them, I nurse them."[45] The work of these pediatric surgeons, performed in less than optimum conditions, suggested a growing need for a specialized hospital for children.

It was not long in coming. Led by Luke Able, many of these professionals pushed for the development of a children's hospital. The dream became reality in 1954 with the opening of the Texas Children's Hospital (TCH). Adjoining St. Luke's Episcopal Hospital, the original 106-

bed facility was a welcome addition to the burgeoning Texas Medical Center complex.[46] Headed by TCH physician-in-chief, Dr. Russell Blattner (1954–1977), hospital staff consisted entirely of members of the Houston Pediatric Society. Many of these pediatricians were specialists, including pediatric anesthesiologists, oncologists, radiologists, pathologists, and surgeons. The idea of creating an entire hospital staffed by physicians specializing in the care of children was a unique approach in a medical community where most pediatric patients remained under the traditional auspices of general practitioners.[47]

As the newly appointed surgeon-in-chief, Luke Able launched the pediatric surgery division at TCH. By 1956, Able was performing between fifteen to twenty pediatric surgeries per week. To help alleviate the heavy caseload, Able collaborated with Baylor College of Medicine to create a residency program in pediatric surgery. The first trainee, Dr. Franklin J. Harberg, ultimately succeeded Able as chief of surgery at Texas Children's. In 1958, surgical pioneer Dr. Benjy Brooks arrived at TCH, where she remained until 1973 when she assumed the role as Division Chair of Pediatrics at UT. Through hard work and dedication Able, Brooks, and Harberg carried pediatric surgery in Houston for the next twenty years.[48]

Richard Andrassy's arrival on the scene in 1985 signaled a new era for pediatric surgery in Houston: a fundamental shift from private practice to full-time academic surgery. "There was really no academic pediatric surgery at the time in Houston," he later recalled. "The private docs in town would cover whatever things had to be done. But there was very low case volume and most of it was transferred to Texas Children's."[49] By assuming the dual chairs of pediatric surgery at UT and M. D. Anderson, Andrassy entered new territory. While his new position sounded good on paper, Andrassy quickly understood that he was practically starting from scratch. His predecessor, Benjy Brooks, had retired from practice in 1982, thus creating a long vacancy. From "a very old office with an old dial phone and a bunch of boxes and dust," Andrassy was put in charge of an empty division. "Theoretically," he noted, "I was Professor and Chief of Pediatric Surgery, but I had no secretary, no nurse, no real office . . . and I was on call every single day because I was it." The situation at M. D. Anderson turned out to be bare bones as well. No pediatric service existed at the hospital, leaving the care of child patients to adult surgeons.

As a result, the hospital lacked many of the basics for pediatric surgery. There was no 4-0 silk for child sutures, no instruments designed for use on children, and no Intensive Care Unit for the young patients. "We did not have any place to put sick kids," Andrassy explained. "I used to have to transfer them over here [Hermann Hospital], operate on them, then transfer them back [to M. D. Anderson]. I spent a lot of hours walking back and forth."[50] Having come from the well-equipped environment of Wilford Hall, Andrassy's early experience in Houston was challenging. The primary task, as Andrassy saw it, involved growth and stability within the division. He purchased needed equipment, established laboratories, and began recruiting faculty. In addition to occupying an endowed chair, Andrassy had at his disposal an endowed professorship position and another fund for visiting professors. In 1987, Dr. Tom Black, a Baylor College of Medicine graduate (1979) who completed pediatric fellowships at Baylor and McGaw Medical Center in Chicago, became the first faculty hire. In September 1991, Dr. Kevin Lally joined Andrassy at UT. "I had decided that I was going to separate from the air force," Lally recalled, "and in looking around for jobs, Rich asked me to look at this job here in Houston."[51] The fundraising expertise of former chair, Benjy Brooks, aided Lally's decision. "There was an endowed professorship that was unfilled . . . That professorship as well as the endowed chair that Rich held at the time was really important. [Brooks] also set up another fund for visiting professors." In retrospect, Lally observed, "All have been very useful to both the faculty and helping us grow."[52]

The creation of a solid residency program in pediatric surgery was another key to departmental success. To do so, Andrassy started from the ground up with general surgery residents. "The second year resident would follow me everywhere," Andrassy recalled, "to Anderson and to Hermann . . . and then little by little," Andrassy observed, "a lot of them got interested in pediatric surgery. When we started getting a fourth year on the service, they had another opportunity to come back and operate with us."[53]

The timing in this instance proved advantageous. Andrassy's efforts to build the UT pediatric surgery program during the late 1980s and early 1990s coincided with a national trend toward subspecialization of general surgery. Traditionally, general surgeons conducted the gamut of surgical procedures, whether thoracic, plastic, vascular, or pediatric. However, the

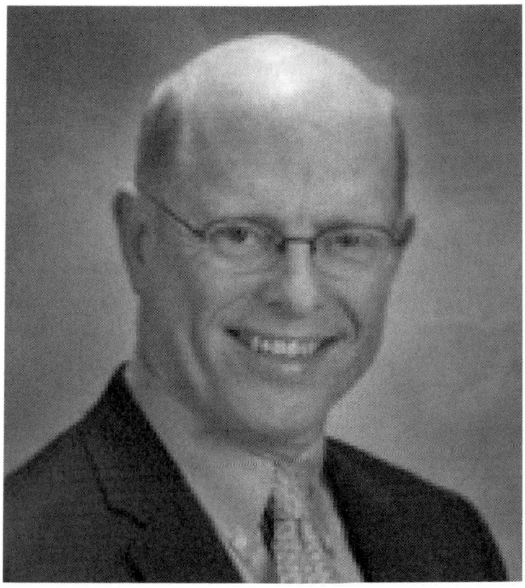

Kevin P. Lally, MD.

rise of surgical specialization over the past two decades had led to better expertise by surgeons focused on many niche areas of surgery, including all areas of surgery for children. Andrassy encouraged the development of this trend within his department. As he worked with general surgical residents, Andrassy stimulated new avenues of exploration through the writing of clinical papers or laboratory work involving various aspects of pediatric surgery. One involved the innovative extracorporeal membrane oxygenation (ECMO) program. Established in 1992 and directed by Dr. Kevin Lally, the program provided excellent exposure to the intricacies of pediatric critical care.[54]

The opening of LBJ Hospital in 1989 provided an additional boost. The high volume caseload among the three hospitals—M. D. Anderson, Hermann, and LBJ—delivered a wealth of surgical training opportunities to UT residents, more than enough to encourage many residents to subspecialize in pediatric surgery. By the early 1990s, Andrassy later noted, UT-Houston ranked third in the United States regarding the number of medical school residents choosing to enter pediatric surgery.[55]

Over the next few years, the pediatric surgery division continued to develop under Andrassy's careful supervision. Then came a sudden change. Having reached the age of sixty-five, Frank Moody stepped down as Chairman of Surgery, thus creating a need for someone to serve as Interim Chairman. Dr. John C. Ribble, dean of the Medical School (1986–1994), approached Andrassy about the job. After almost ten years at UT, Andrassy had built a solid reputation as a pediatric surgeon. But it was his business acumen that had particular appeal to Ribble. "I was building up Pediatric Surgery well at the time," Andrassy explained, "and this was the time when we thought we were going to go to capitation. I had learned a lot about managed care. I had decided to study it mainly so that I could try to help build the Pediatric Surgery referral base." Ribble understood the exceptional value of a surgeon trained to navigate the intricacies of administrative finance.[56]

On August 15, 1994, Andrassy became Interim Chair of Surgery at UT-Houston while the school conducted a nationwide search for a full-time chair. None of the candidates, however, seemed to possess Andrassy's level of business expertise. According to Andrassy, "Several of the people that came to look at the job knew me and even made a comment to [Ribble], 'Why don't you make him the Chair, because he understands?'"[57] Nevertheless, Andrassy was surprised when, after nine months of searching for Moody's replacement, Dean Ribble offered him the job. "I thought he was going to tell me [the search committee] had made a selection and thanks for my help. Instead, the committee asked me to consider [staying in the position permanently]."[58]

It was an exceptional offer. In those days few pediatric surgeons had ever served as university chairs. "Some department chairs questioned how a pediatrician could become head of surgery, not understanding that we actually train in general surgery first," Andrassy later observed. The fact that Andrassy kept one foot in the world of adult surgery undoubtedly advanced his prospects. "I was still doing some adult sarcomas at the county hospital and at M. D. Anderson. It gave me some credibility that a surgeon that takes care of children could also take care of adults."[59] In May, 1995, Andrassy advanced to the chairmanship and appointed Kevin Lally to succeed him as division chair. By this time, Dr. Lally had built a national reputation, and others were courting him to be division head.

Many challenges awaited Andrassy as he assumed leadership. Continued growth within the Department of Surgery demanded the expansion of its academic, clinical, and research base. Success depended upon the recruitment of additional faculty, the tightening up of fiscal policies and

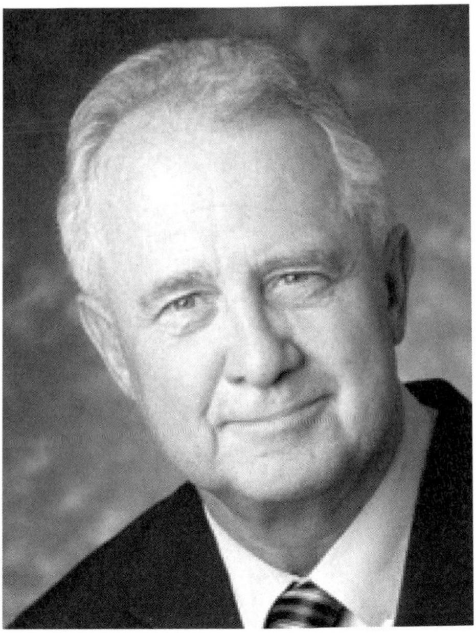

Richard J. Andrassy, MD, the third Chairman of the Department of Surgery.

procedures, and the development of surgical specialty programs at affiliated hospitals. It was a tall order for Andrassy, but several factors worked in his favor. His reputation in the medical school as a good doctor provided Andrassy the sustained support of established colleagues including, among others, Drs. Dudrick, Moody, Parks, and Kahan. He also possessed a simple management philosophy which he explained, stating: "If I could hire really good people, get them the resources they needed, and then get out of their way, the department would do well, and by reflection, I would look good too."[60] During his tenure as Chair, Andrassy recruited, among other top talent, Dr. Charles S. Cox, UT Distinguished Professor of Pediatric Surgery and innovator in stem cell research, and Dr. Erik B. Wilson, current Director of the Division of Elective General Surgery and specialist in minimally invasive surgery. As a result, Andrassy professed, "I have been very fortunate that the people that I have hired have all had good work ethic and have done a good job building not only a clinical but a research base."[61]

A clear example of Andrassy's early administrative skill can be seen in the restructuring of the Trauma and Critical Care service at Hermann

Hospital. By the mid-1990s, the unit at Hermann had become the busiest trauma center in the world. However, no differentiation existed within the trauma service regarding levels of acute care, causing trauma surgeons to become overwhelmed. "When you were on trauma call, you would take care of everything," Andrassy explained. "If somebody came in with an appendix, and you are in there taking care of gunshot wounds, you do not have time to go do that appendectomy. When you were done doing all the gunshot wounds, then you would do that." As a result, "the patient sits around for days, and the docs are mad and the patients are mad."[62] Such scenarios also hampered the training of residents. The question at hand involved finding an effective way to expedite the care of hospital patients with non-traumatic surgical conditions.

The solution involved the establishment of an acute care surgery program that would further define and bring into focus the trauma and critical care services. Under this model, acute care surgery would be organized by the following specialties: emergency general surgery (EGS, including appendectomies, perforated ulcers, etc.), trauma and critical care (ICU care of the patient), and a few years later, burns. Each specialty had a separate service with doctors on call and residents reporting to a separate chief. However, since they are all interrelated, each specialty remained under the umbrella of Acute Care Surgery. As opposed to smaller hospitals where surgeons on call handle whatever emergency comes through the hospital doors, UT surgeons primarily remained within their specialty.[63]

While the endeavor lacked initial funding resources and support, Andrassy put his weight behind it and implemented a trial run on July 1, 1996. "I took call myself [for] nine days to see if it was going to work," said Andrassy. "It started working great. The residents loved it. The patients loved it. The referring doctors loved it."[64] Shortly afterward, the Department of Surgery acquired a grant to finance the operation. The next priority involved the creation of an acute care surgery team.

To build it, Andrassy recruited Dr. Fred Moore, a young, talented associate professor of surgery at the University of Colorado Health Science Center in Denver. It was a good choice. Over the following decade, Moore effectively fostered development of the Division of Acute Care Surgery through administration of the trauma center grant, the creation of a burn unit, and the establishment of academic fellowships in the areas of research, trauma, burns, and critical care. In 2007, Moore left the department to become Chief of the Division of Surgical Critical Care and Acute care at the Methodist Hospital.[65]

The following year, Andrassy welcomed Moore's replacement, renowned military surgeon Dr. John B. Holcomb. Over a twenty-three-year career in the United States Army, Holcomb earned the reputation as one of the military's top trauma surgeons. As Chief of the Division of Acute Care Surgery and current Vice Chair of the Department of Surgery, Holcomb continues to advance the mission through the further development of surgical care groups, fellowships, and the establishment of a Center for Translational Injury Research.[66]

A pediatric trauma program developed in tandem with the Acute Care Services division at Hermann. In 1997, the UT Pediatric Surgical Team partnered with Children's Memorial Hermann Hospital and the Children's Cancer Hospital at M. D. Anderson to create a specialized trauma unit for pediatric patients. Equipped to meet the needs of patients with conditions ranging from minor injuries and illnesses to major trauma, the Galtney Trauma and Emergency Center was the first Level I pediatric trauma center established in the Texas Gulf Coast region. "The integration with Children's Memorial Hermann helped us deliver really outstanding care," observed pediatric surgical division chair, Kevin Lally. For instance, he recalled the first fetal surgical procedure performed by the UT team in 1999. "I was delivering a baby with a really big neck mass," Lally recalled. "That procedure is you put the mom to sleep, open the uterus, expose the baby—but there is still placental support—and establish an airway. That was the big issue. Before, you would use the umbilical cord flow. Once we effectively established the airway, we clamped the cord, delivered the baby, and moved the baby with a tracheostomy in place."[67] Such successes spurred the reputation of the center and UT surgeons. Directed by UT Professor of Pediatric Surgery, Charles Cox, the center currently administers around-the-clock care to over 18,000 children in emergency situations each year.[68]

Throughout his years as UT Chair of Surgery, Richard Andrassy has encouraged the efforts of all divisions within the department. However, perhaps no group has benefited more from Andrassy's sound experience and long-term vision than the Division of Pediatric Surgery, which became

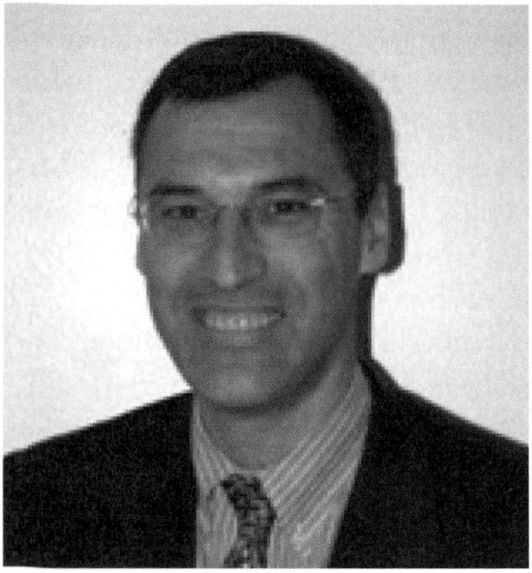

Charles S. Cox, Jr., MD.

a separate department of the Medical School in 2007. "This department would not exist without Rich Andrassy's support," claimed Lally. "He was a pioneer."[69] Having started with just Andrassy in 1985, the Division of Pediatric Surgery has grown into a thriving department of thirty-three faculty members spread among five divisions: general and thoracic pediatric surgery, pediatric neurosurgery, pediatric plastic and craniofacial surgery, pediatric cardiovascular surgery, and pediatric trauma. Resident and fellowship training programs also continue the ongoing quest for medical excellence.[70] Important departmental achievements include the creation of a successful Extracorporeal Membrane Oxygenation program (ECMO) and the development of a Level I pediatric trauma center. Dr. Charles Cox served as the principal investigator for the first trial on stem cells for traumatic brain injury. In March of 2012, UT pediatric surgeons comprised the first team in Texas to conduct a fetal repair of myelomeningocele (open spinal cord) outside of a child.[71] Clinical research spearheaded by Andrassy has also created an impact. From early projects involving enteral feeding to cancer surgery and studies regarding neurofibromatosis, each endeavor has brought fresh focus to the field of pediatric surgery.

In 2010, he made another advance in the development of an exciting, new surgical procedure to correct a rare but debilitating and dangerous birth defect. Each year, approximately one in 4,000 infants is born with an omphalocele, a physical manifestation that occurs when the fetus' abdominal wall fails to close properly. The baby is born with several internal organs growing in a thin sack outside the body. The condition could be "devastating," Andrassy observed. "These kids just have skin over their liver and intestines, so they cannot play sports or do anything normal children do."[72] Some omphaloceles are small enough to be corrected shortly after birth by tucking the organs back into the body and closing the abdominal wall. In the case of larger defects, surgeons traditionally wait until the patient is ten to twelve years of age before attempting to reconstruct the abdominal wall. At that point, multiple operations are required to pull the muscle fascia over the organs.[73]

Andrassy had an idea. In his work with adult patients, he had utilized a new surgical technique called "component separation." The technique involves separating the top layer of three muscles—the external oblique, the internal oblique, and the transversal—freeing the muscles to slide toward the midline, in accordion-like fashion. A piece of biologic mesh is then inserted underneath to help reinforce and close the abdomen. Andrassy found this procedure highly effective in the cases of over 125 adults needing hernia repairs or abdominal reconstructive surgery. Perhaps, Andrassy thought, the procedure could be "modified down" for children. "We have had some very complicated cases, such as a man who had thirty-eight previous operations, who did quite well after a component separation," Andrassy reasoned. "I started wondering if we could do it in children. The hesitation was always that it was unclear if there was enough musculature to do it."[74] However, if the procedure worked, pediatric patients with a large omphalocele would only face one operation rather than the multiple ones usually required to stretch the muscles and skin over the abdomen.[75]

UT surgeons initially tried the operation on a nine-year-old with a sizable omphalocele. It was a success. Andrassy's team conducted successive operations on other children ranging in age from two years old to nine, and then finally, a nine-month-old infant. "Each [procedure] turned out nicely," Andrassy recalled. "Then we said, 'Why can't we try this in a newborn?' Wouldn't it be better to try to do the repair then instead of waiting until they were older?"[76] In time, Andrassy effectively performed a component separation on a five-day-old newborn. He later learned to his surprise that his tiny patient was the youngest baby in the world to receive the component separation surgery. "I realized nobody had done newborns before," Andrassy admitted. "If you are dumb enough to not know that people have not done it, you just do it and then there you go."[77]

To date, the long-term effects of this innovative technique are unclear. Yet, Andrassy and fellow pediatric surgeons remain highly optimistic. As a result of undergoing component separation surgery, infant and very young patients can move their legs well, roll on their stomachs, and crawl easily across the floor. Patients a few years older can do sit-ups and many other physical activities. Other benefits are also evident. According to Andrassy, this surgical procedure, one that most pediatric surgeons can "easily learn," would further enhance the ability of UT surgeons to care for children with giant omphaloceles, open abdomens from trauma, or from other life-threatening complications.[78]

Recent improvements pertaining to abdominal wall reconstruction techniques exemplify the beauty of pediatric surgery. "There is always some new focus that you can move to," Andrassy observed, that incorporates new opportunities for teaching, training, and research.[79] Over the past century pediatric surgeons have contributed immeasurably to the field. However, profound developments over the past three decades have made so much more possible. Critical advances in anesthesia enable pediatric surgeons to conduct major surgery on tiny infants who traditionally had no chance of survival. The development of minimal access surgery has stimulated the invention of surgical equipment sized compatibly to infants and small children. Moreover, the growing emphasis on subspecialization has vastly contributed to the expansion of programs and initiatives related to all areas of pediatric surgery. It has been a time of monumental change, to which Andrassy has been a witness. More importantly, as former head of the Medical School's Division of Pediatric Surgery and current Chairman of the Department of Surgery, Andrassy has overseen a cutting edge participation in the revolution. During his tenure as Chair of Surgery, he has encouraged his team to explore innovative new ideas through research and to stay in the forefront of both developing and adopting new surgical techniques.

Over time, Andrassy's predecessors as chair—Stan Dudrick and Frank Moody—set a precedent for establishing the department's reputation for excellence and innovation. Following in their footsteps, Rich Andrassy raised the bar and brought his own formidable leadership skills to the department. Today, The University of Texas Medical School at Houston Department of Surgery is one of the top surgical programs in the country. None of this would surprise either Dudrick or Moody, both of whom recognized Andrassy's talent and had a hand in bringing him to Houston. As the longest-serving current chair of surgery in the country, Andrassy faced many administrative challenges during his years in the position. At times, this has meant creating new surgical divisions within the department or spinning off some divisions into new departments of their own. His ability to adapt quickly in the often rapidly changing milieu that is the world of modern academic surgery has served him well and created a professional environment in which the surgical divisions within the department would continue to thrive and achieve remarkable success for years to come.

CHAPTER 7

Evolution in Trauma

Acute Care, Oral and Maxillofacial, and Plastic Surgery

At the time Dr. Richard J. Andrassy took over as interim chair of the Department of Surgery in 1994, the department was in the midst of a cycle of change in its structure and organization. Some of the original divisions had broken out into separate surgical departments during the Moody era, including Neurosurgery, Orthopaedic Surgery, and Otorhinolaryngology. During Andrassy's tenure as department chair, Cardiothoracic and Vascular Surgery followed in 1999 and Pediatric Surgery in 2007. Under Andrassy's leadership, the surgical divisions have continued to evolve and mature, enhancing the department's reputation and making it one of the largest practice programs in the country.

One area in which the department has been a national leader almost from its inception and throughout its history is Trauma Service. Early on, this unit continued to grow in size and expertise, with Dr. Ronald Fischer directing the trauma program and Dr. Red Duke serving as Medical Director of the Hermann Hospital Life Flight. By the early 1980s, Hermann Hospital's (Memorial Hermann—TMC after merger in July 1997) Life Flight program had grown to include a fleet of five helicopters, which helped to make the Trauma Service the largest and most active in the United States and earned an NIH grant to fund a Trauma Research Center. The steadily increasing patient load in the emergency room at Memorial Hermann–TMC and the development of new surgical technologies during the 1990s all contributed to a need to change the way surgeons cared for patients in the emergency room. In response, Andrassy, along with Dr. Fred Moore, developed the concept of acute care surgery as an umbrella program that would include but also distinguish between emergency trauma cases and other types of emergency surgeries. The program immediately showed benefits for both surgeons and patients, and Andrassy quickly took steps to make it a separate service with doctors on call, separate residents, and a separate chief, but remaining a Division in the Department of Surgery. One offshoot of this reorganization was that the Division of Emergency Medicine was spun off into its own separate department. Today, the Department of Emergency Medicine is headed by Department Chair James J. McCarthy, MD, and maintains a curriculum designed to provide residents with emergency department experience by working with highly skilled emergency doctors. And since the Division of Acute Care Surgery was organized in 1996, it has continued to develop in technical expertise, improved patient care, and outreach into the community. The division now includes Trauma, Critical Care, Emergency General Surgery, and Burns.[1]

Part of the success of Acute Care Surgery is due to Andrassy successfully recruiting a highly experienced and renowned military trauma surgeon, Dr. John B. Holcomb, to join the faculty and serve as Division Director. Holcomb, who replaced Fred Moore, was also appointed Director of the Center for Translational Injury Research (CTIR). John B. Holcomb was literally born into the US Army at Fort Benning, Georgia, where his father was stationed at the time, but he spent most of his youth in Fort Smith, Arkansas, a town of about 60,000. He recalled wanting to become a doctor from a very early age. "There is a picture of me when I was six years old with a stethoscope, listening to my brother's heart," he recalled. "I always liked science, and I worked as an operating room technician as a summer job in Fort Smith. I really liked surgery and liked being the operating room technician." He went to Centenary College in Shreveport, Louisiana, where he received a Bachelor of Science degree in biology, graduating with honors in 1981. But when he received his letter of acceptance into medical school, Holcomb realized he had no way to pay the tuition. However, the armed services had a scholarship program called the Health Professions Scholarship Program (HPSP) available for medical students in return for their service in the military after graduation. Although the air force and navy also had scholarship programs, Holcomb chose the army entirely because his father served in that branch of the armed forces. Holcomb earned his MD from the University of Arkansas Medical School in 1985 and subsequently entered the US Army, where he completed his general surgery internship in 1986 and his general surgery residency in 1991, both at the William Beaumont Army Medical Center in El Paso, Texas. During 1990, a colleague approached Holcomb to gauge his interest about participating in a special assignment. This led to him joining the United States Special Operations Command (USSOCOM) in 1991 and being deployed with them for nine years supporting US Special Forces including the Navy SEALs and Army Rangers. In 1993, Holcombe found himself in Somalia supporting Task Force Ranger, a Joint Special Operations Task Force (JSOTF) assigned to capture Somali warlord Gen. Mohammed Farah Aideed, along with several others, and to turn over the captives to the United Nations forces. Their raid on October 3–4, 1993, became known as the "Black Hawk Down" incident. "It was my first real experience with combat casualty care as a surgeon," said Holcomb. "I had first taken care of combat casualties out of Panama in 1989 as a fourth-year resident when I was rotating in the thoracic service at Brooke Army Medical Center in San Antonio. But as a surgeon in 1993, I was in the 'Black Hawk Down' incident." All of this had a profound impact on Holcomb, who then decided to remain in the army to do research on developing more effective ways to prevent death from hemorrhaging in the event of traumatic injury.[2]

From 1991 to 2008, Holcomb served in numerous military posts and rose to the rank of colonel. He was awarded several decorations for service, including the Bronze Star, the Honorary Medal for Combat Surgical Care, and in 2005, the Department of the Army Research and Development Achievement Award for Leadership Excellence. From 2002 to 2008, Dr. Holcomb served as both Commander of the US Army Institute of Surgical Research and as Trauma Consultant for the Army Surgeon General, where he led the only Surgical Research Laboratory in the Department of Defense. In 2008, Holcomb joined The University of Texas Health Science Center at Houston as Professor of Surgery and Head of the Division of Acute Care Surgery. "The elements were already in the department," said Holcomb. "Dr. Andrassy allowed us to reorganize some things, and we brought the burn center into the Division of Acute Care Surgery. We also had Emergency General Surgery, EGS

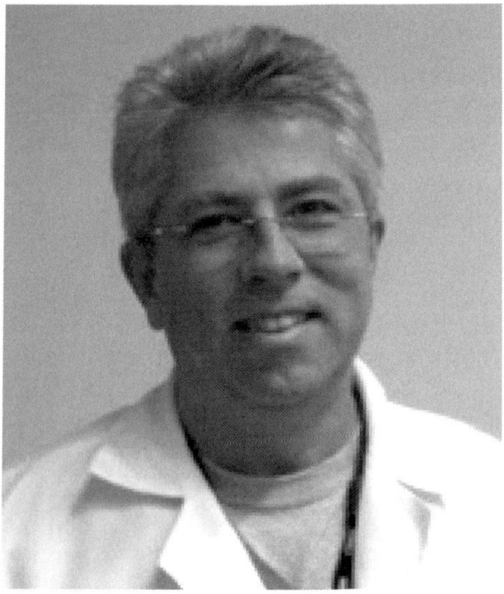

John B. Holcomb, MD.

we call it—appendectomies, perforated ulcers, diverticulitis—whatever emergency operation the general surgeons do are done by that group. We had the trauma group that does the trauma surgery and then we have a surgical critical care group that does the ICU care of the patient. So, those four sections are now the Division of Acute Care Surgery." In order to enhance training in Acute Care Surgery, the division developed a number of fellowships including a Burn Fellowship, a Critical Care Fellowship, a Trauma Fellowship, and a Research Fellowship.[3]

Soon after joining the faculty, Holcomb became the Director of the Center for Translational Injury Research. This is a university-wide center that takes research findings from the laboratory and translates them to clinical application in caring for patients. Medical research has changed dramatically and become very specialized in the past forty years. Today, much of the actual research work is conducted by PhD-level scientists who focus only on laboratory studies. Then it is the clinicians who take the next step by "translating" the discoveries and quality initiatives from the research laboratory for testing and application in the clinical setting. John Holcomb embraced this new role enthusiastically, as it gave him the opportunity to continue research he had begun during his years in the army and also provided an application for some of his findings. "The Center for Translational Injury Research is taking good ideas from the lab and doing clinical studies and then implementing the result of those clinical studies into clinical practice," explained Holcomb. "Translating the good ideas from the basic science world—what we should do for patients—into well-designed clinical studies that they can document with Level-1 evidence: that is what the Center for Translational Injury Research does."[4]

Trauma care and research have been among the hallmarks at The University of Texas Medical School and at Memorial Hermann–TMC since the inception of the Department of Surgery in 1974. With so much expertise in what has become the nation's busiest trauma center, on May 29, 2012, officials from Memorial Hermann Healthcare System announced the creation of the Texas Trauma Institute at Memorial Hermann–Texas Medical Center and named Dr. John Holcomb as Director. The goal of the new institute, the first of its kind in Texas, is to dedicate clinical resources and research to improve outcomes for both adult and pediatric trauma patients. The institute would continue the legacy in Houston trauma medicine pioneered by Dr. James "Red" Duke and would be based on the long-term affiliation with the Medical School. In a press release, Holcomb stated: "With trauma injury projected to be the leading cause of death worldwide by the year 2020, the Institute will provide us with a unique opportunity to move research from the laboratory to the bedside. The Institute will be a wonderful catalyst for driving innovations in trauma care by providing us with the necessary data that can help improve the survival and recovery rates of trauma victims, not only in the Houston region, but throughout the United States." The Texas Trauma Institute would offer exceptional care and provide a full range of services and resources to both adult and pediatric trauma patients, including Memorial Hermann's Life Flight and Houston's only certified burn center. Preliminary plans called for the trauma center to be housed in its own structure adjacent to the main hospital.[5] On April 16, 2014, Memorial Hermann Health System unveiled plans for a $650 million expansion and renovation project at its Texas Medical Center hospital. Approved by the Memorial Hermann Health System board in March, the plans included a new patient care building that would house most of the hospital's trauma and specialty intensive care units, adding 160 beds, twenty-four new operating rooms, and sixteen new emergency room bays. Construction was to begin on the four-year project during the summer 2014 and also included more parking, new loading docks, and other needed updates to the hospital's infrastructure.[6]

Holcomb anticipated that the new building housing the Institute, connecting directly to Memorial Hermann Hospital, would be the place where all the trauma patients received care. The notion of improving care by bringing trauma patients together in one area rather than scattered all over the hospital also means bringing many medical specialists and disciplines together in the same space. The concept required a lot of reorganizing and presented both opportunities and challenges. Holcomb acknowledged that while one of the appealing things about working in trauma is that it is an inherently multidisciplinary field requiring neurosurgery, orthopedics, ophthalmology, psychiatry, emergency medicine, anesthesia, general surgery, and many more specialists to provide care; conversely the same multidisciplinary aspects also present many organizational challenges. But about 25 percent of patients at Memorial Hermann are trauma victims, and with the hospital being the largest trauma center in the United States, the opportunity to become a leader in trauma research and patient care could not be ignored.

The Center for Disease Control and Prevention estimates that trauma is the leading cause of death in America for ages one to forty-four. Consequently, because it afflicts primarily young people, one of the many tragic results of trauma is its cost in life-years lost in the United States, estimated to be four times that of heart disease and cancer. For example, if a trauma victim dies at age twenty, one could presume that the patient has lost perhaps fifty to sixty years of life. Because some thirty million people get injured every year—about one-tenth of the US population—the resulting loss of years lived and the productivity that might have been part of them is huge. This loss of so many lives due to trauma injuries added a sense of urgency and purpose as Holcomb developed plans for the new trauma center. Education and prevention would be part of the mix, along with research and developing new protocols for patient care. Holcomb anticipated reaching out to experts in the School of Public Health, the School of Nursing, and the Medical School, and also to local medics through Life Flight, the Houston Fire Department, and to contacts in the military, Special Operations EMS, and FBI units in the area.

It is not beyond imagination that this could become a national center, one day making Houston as renowned for trauma care and research as it has been for research in cardiology and heart surgery. "We are the biggest trauma center in the United States already, in the biggest medical center in the country," said Holcomb. "We already have the [patients] and this opportunity really is something special."[7]

One of the first applications to come from the new Texas Trauma Institute was the wide-spread use of modern tourniquets by Houston-area emergency responders. In February 2014, the Memorial Hermann Hospital Texas Trauma Institute announced that it would donate 5,000 first aid kits containing combat tourniquets to the Houston Police Department. The idea came from Holcomb's experience and research as an army trauma surgeon in Baghdad. Holcomb coauthored a study that showed the benefits of using tourniquets in combat and that when properly utilized they improved survival without increasing complications. In a press statement, Holcomb said, "The significance of the use of tourniquets and gauze on the battlefield is the main lesson to save lives in the civilian community." The objective of the tourniquet program is to provide all Houston patrol officers with two tourniquets and gauze. Police officers would be trained in how to use the kits with the goal that by 2015, all uniformed officers would have the skills and equipment to use these emergency kits, followed by training for investigators and other nonuniformed officers. Houston would be joining the ranks of other major cities including Dallas, Philadelphia, and Los Angeles that have equipped their police forces with similar emergency medical supplies. Holcomb viewed the implementation of tourniquets in the city as being a major step forward. "Tourniquets were not being used in Houston or at UT when I got here," stated Holcomb. "Based on my experience in the military, we put tourniquets on Life Flight; we put tourniquets in the emergency department, and through the Regional Advisory Council purchased thousands of tourniquets and put them on the ambulances. Tourniquets are now a normal practice in Houston."[8]

In addition to the tourniquet program for HPD, Holcombe and Dr. Red Duke, Medical Director for the Memorial Hermann Life Flight program, collaborated on several innovative new therapies for trauma patients. "We worked together on the implementation of tourniquets and monitors," said Holcomb. "We put blood and blood products on the helicopter one year ago, so we were one of two helicopter services (the other is at Mayo Clinic) that have plasma and red cells on the helicopter." During the first year with plasma and red cells on the helicopter, Life Flight EMTs treated over 100 patients, significantly improving patient outcomes. This continuing focus on improving trauma care as manifest by the establishment of the Division of Acute Care Surgery, the Center for Translational Injury Research, and then the Texas Trauma Center, soon led to implementation of new procedures for seriously injured patients. "I think the most important advance is that we have implemented the resuscitation concepts that came out of the military," said Holcomb. "We have a large number of bleeding patients, and our resuscitation techniques have been the biggest determinant of improved outcome in our patients." [9]

In addition to developing new procedures, CTIR has conducted extensive studies and published its findings on coagulation, bleeding, and resuscitation. The Center has documented outcomes of these changes that include markedly improved mortality in the sickest patients (by 60 percent over the last four years) and in all 6,000 trauma admissions, patient survival improved by 20 percent. "Those are significant improvements," observed Holcomb. "I think that is our biggest contribution right now." CTIR also has leveraged its NIH and Department of Defense (DOD) funding for prospective randomized studies, implemented new procedures and lessons learned in the military, and led several multicenter studies across the country and in Toronto.[10]

Thus, what began with the decision years ago by Drs. Dudrick, Duke, and Copeland to take call and begin improving professional services in the emergency room of an aging, tired hospital set a pattern for bold innovation in the future and led to the Memorial Hermann–TMC emergency room becoming the busiest and one of the most renowned trauma centers in the country. The success of the newly organized division of Acute Care Surgery is based, in part, on the collaborative, multidisciplinary nature of the program. Among the various divisions in the Department of Surgery that often are called upon to treat trauma patients who arrive with severe head injuries are the surgeons of the Division of Oral and Maxillofacial Surgery, which also is a division of the UT School of Dentistry. "But since their residents rotate with us and are such an integral part of taking care of our trauma patients—all the head and neck and injuries—they have always been a part of the Department [of Surgery]," said Andrassy. "And it has always been a quality group of docs there." The staff of Oral and Maxillofacial Surgery of the School of Dentistry supports the Division of Oral and Maxillofacial Surgery in the Department of Surgery and provides care to patients in the Texas Medical Center. The Division has a four-year residency program based at the Dental Branch, with sixteen residents who rotate through Memorial Hermann–TMC, Ben Taub General Hospital, Methodist Hospital, and the Michael E. DeBakey Veterans Administration Medical Center. Residents gain experience in oral and maxillofacial surgery and in providing care for surgical trauma patients at Memorial Hermann Hospital.[11]

The UTHealth School of Dentistry was one of the original institutions of the Texas Medical Center and has its origins in the Texas Dental College, which was founded in 1905 as a proprietary school. By the early 1930s, the Great Depression had taken a toll on the dental college, resulting in low enrollment and financial problems. In 1932, the board of trustees recruited Dr. Frederick C. Elliott, dean at the University of Tennessee, Memphis, School of Dentistry, to take over as dean of the Texas Dental College. Elliott reinvigorated the Texas Dental College and eventually succeeded in his efforts to bring the school into The University of Texas System. On September 1, 1943, the Texas Dental College officially became The University of Texas School of Dentistry. With the end of World War II in 1945, the Dental Branch began expanding its programs. Three years later, in May 1948, the school appointed Dr. Edward C. Hinds as the first Chairman of the Department of Oral Surgery, making it the first formal oral surgery training program in Texas. Hinds had earned his medical degree from Baylor College of Medicine (before it moved to Houston) and his dental degree at Baylor College of Dentistry in Dallas. Since the establishment of the oral surgery program in 1948, there have been three chairs of the department: Edward C. Hinds (1948–1983), John C. Helfrick (1984–2000) and Mark E. K. Wong (2000–present). The residency program has matured over the years from a two-year program in the beginning to parallel programs of either four or six years, with residents in the six-year program also earning a medical

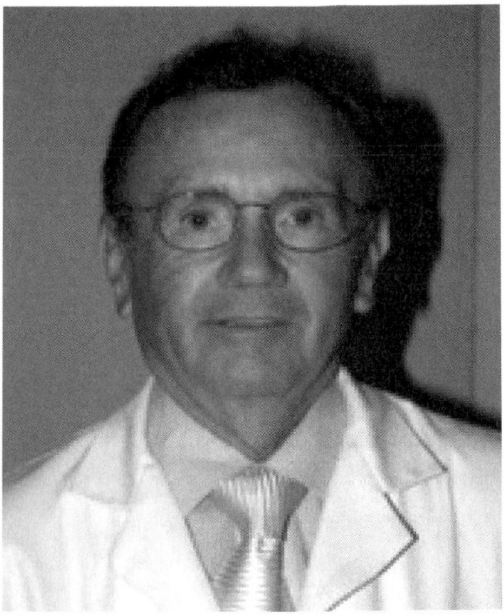

Donald H. Parks, MD.

degree from The University of Texas Medical School. Today, the training program is the largest and one of the highest rated in the country. Residents who have completed the program are in practice throughout Texas and the United States. Their success has also made them good ambassadors of the School of Dentistry, enhancing its reputation and making the program "one of the most sought-after residency programs for oral and maxillofacial training in the world."[12]

In addition to the Division of Oral and Maxillofacial Surgery, Plastic and Reconstructive Surgery also has a key role in the multidisciplinary milieu that comprises Acute Care Surgery and the trauma center. As discussed previously, Dr. Donald H. Parks had joined the Department of Surgery in 1982. At the time, Hermann Hospital had a small burn center that had been established in 1979 under the direction of Hermann Hospital's CEO, Bill Smith, and Drs. James Smith and David E. Beesinger of the Department of Surgery. Basically, they had sectioned off an area of the Robertson Wing of Hermann Hospital, put up a sign, and called it the Institute for Thermal Injuries. This original burn center was a fairly small area comprised of about twelve patient rooms in the south wing on the seventh floor of the Robertson Pavilion. By the time Parks arrived in 1982, Smith had left and Beesinger was running the burn center. Beesinger had joined the department in 1979 and served as director of the burn center for four years until 1983, when he left Houston to go into private practice in Bryan/College Station, thus leaving Parks in charge of the Burn Center. In 1985, Dr. William Reilly, chair of Plastic and Reconstructive Surgery, left the medical school to go into private practice, and Parks was appointed to Division Chair.[13]

During the years after the burn center first opened, Hermann Hospital had done some renovations and created an intensive care unit in the burn center. "It was starting to look a little bit more like a burn center but still not quite," Parks recalled. "The patients were taken from that wing of the hospital on elevators down to operating rooms a long way away and then wheeled back. We had problems with patients getting in trouble in the elevators, and it was less than ideal." During the ensuing years, Parks worked closely with Steve Dunn of the John S. Dunn Foundation (established in 1977), and with officials at Hermann Hospital in a continuing process of upgrading the burn facility into a comprehensive burn center. Steve Dunn had been seriously burned and he had been treated by a very famous Houston plastic surgeon, Dr. Thomas D. Cronin (Cronin and Dr. Frank Gerow had performed the first breast implant procedure in 1962). In 1986, the Dunn Foundation provided a major gift to The University of Texas and established the Dr. Thomas D. Cronin Chair in Plastic Surgery, with Parks being appointed to that chair. In addition to the endowment for the Cronin Chair, the Dunn family expressed an interest in burn care and in developing a more comprehensive burn unit. They worked with the hospital to provide more modifications and upgrades in the Burn Center and during that period of time began discussions with Parks about creating a first-class burn center that would rank with the best in the country. Houston's population continued to grow, and with no other major burn facility in the city, the need for a comprehensive burn center was significant. The John S. Dunn Foundation offered to provide a significant part of the funds to be combined with support from Hermann Hospital.

During the next few years, Parks, the Dunn Foundation, and officials from Hermann Hospital engaged in a long series of meetings, planning sessions, and discussions about what the new burn center should look like, the number of patient beds it would need, and all the details related to equipping and staffing a major burn center. The process dragged on, in part, because the Hermann Hospital administration had changed a few times, and then in 1997, Hermann Hospital merged with the Memorial Health Care System, becoming Memorial Hermann Hospital (known today as Memorial Hermann–TMC). The end result was a plan for a modern, state-of-the-art burn center with about fourteen patient beds. But when Parks saw the final plan as proposed by Hermann Hospital officials, he was extremely disappointed. The center would be situated again in the Robertson Pavilion, but in a space with few windows. "It was dark and dingy and, to me, it was depressing," said Parks. "The last thing we wanted was to have a burn center that was depressing, since patients were so sick; the last thing they needed were dark quarters." By chance, Parks bumped into Dr. Lloyd Gregory, medical director of the Dunn Foundation, while shopping at a local clothing store. Gregory inquired as to the status of the Burn Center planning, and Parks decided on the spot to be up front about the proposed facility. "I don't think we should do it, because we are getting some real estate that we don't want," he told Gregory. "I explained about the location and the dinginess, the darkness, and the depressing geography of the proposed new unit." Gregory's response was, "If that is the way you feel, we will either do something about it or we are not going to do it."[14]

Parks now worried that maybe he had spoken out of turn, but as he recalled later, events moved quickly after his conversation with Gregory. Within the next two days, officials at Hermann rethought the original plans and designated a beautiful section on the eighth floor of the relatively new Jones wing, a bright, cheery area with big windows looking over Fannin Street towards Rice University. Many additional meetings followed, and Parks had an opportunity to have input into the design. "A burn center has to be very carefully designed, because you have very sick patients—many of them dying—and you also have patients that are getting better and getting ready to go home," said Parks. "Everybody is in the same place, but there is dignity involved." It posed a real design dilemma with many aspects to be considered in the process, including care planning, special tubs, tanks, and showers. The final design included a gradation from patients who were being treated for minor burns or getting ready to go home to facilities for patients needing critical care. The

John S. Dunn Sr. Burn Center opened in 2003 on the eighth floor of the Jones Pavilion at Memorial Hermann–Texas Medical Center, a collaborative effort between Memorial Hermann–TMC and the UT Health division of Acute Care Surgery. The center has fourteen beds for acute inpatient care, facilities for physical therapy, occupational therapy, and wound care hydrotherapy, and is the only certified comprehensive burn center in Houston. The Burn Center provides the entire continuum of care including critical care, acute inpatient care, burn reconstruction and scar management, and rehabilitation for patients with burn injuries, inhalation injury, and various skin disorders including Stevens-Johnson Syndrome and Toxic Epidermal Necrolysis. In addition to its state-of-art facility in the Jones Pavilion, the Burn Center has an outpatient clinic located across Fannin Street in the UTHealth Professional Building (formerly the Hermann Professional Building).[15]

Over the years, Parks treated many children with burn injuries and saw a special need in his young patients. In 1986, he organized Camp Janus, a burn camp for children. The camp brought together supporters and volunteers from the Houston Fire Department and Hermann Hospital. One of Parks's first patients, John Tartaglia, donated the initial funds to help get the camp started. This generous gift led to the Camp Janus Fund, a 501(c)(3) that is part of the Memorial Hermann Fund today. Over the years, Parks found many people and philanthropic foundations that were willing to help support the camp. "We perpetuated the camp based on donations from all kinds of people and patients," said Parks. Years ago, the Children's Miracle Network Telethon was a contributor, and Parks also found several attorneys who had settled cases for clients—usually those who had suffered burn accidents—who donated some of their proceeds to the fund.[16]

The camp provides a three-day weekend recreational, therapeutic, and educational experience for children from Texas or nearby, aged five through eighteen, who have recovered or are recovering from burns. The Camp Janus weekend is completely free for children and includes local transportation from Houston and Galveston. Memorial Hermann has worked with the camp in numerous ways including help with transportation, staff volunteers, and even sending one of the Life Flight helicopters to make a guest appearance. Parks recalled that the first camp out in La

Grange, Texas, was very basic in its amenities (no air conditioning) compared with facilities at the present site, Camp-For-All, located near Lake Somerville. Camp-For-All was established in the late 1990s with funds from several philanthropists including the Dunn Foundation and the late John O'Quinn. The camp serves children with all manner of physical and health challenges including burns, cancer, diabetes, and hemophilia. Campers have an opportunity to enjoy all kinds of activities, depending upon their condition. For the burn patients, there is one counselor assigned to each child as they enjoy swimming, fishing, canoeing, horses and other animals, and games and entertainment. "They get out there and nobody cares that faces may be horribly burned or about loss of ears, or a nose gone—that does not seem to matter," said Parks. "They play and it is just a great recovery system for the kids. It is only three days, but it makes a difference to a lot of them." Among the camp's donors are the Houston Fire Fighters Burned Children's Fund, the Wind and Fire Motorcycle Club, and the Junior League of Houston.[17]

After establishing the new burn center and creating Camp Janus for children, Dr. Parks and the Division of Plastic Surgery continued to manage the Burn Center until Parks stepped down as the Burn Center Medical Director in 2010. "At this time, I have actually removed myself from the burn world simply because I could not stay up all night anymore," said Parks during an interview in 2012. During the past thirty years since Dr. Parks first arrived at the Medical School, the Division of Plastic and Reconstructive Surgery has grown in size and scope and matured into one of the key participants in providing trauma care, a component of the multi-disciplinary Acute Care Surgery program. The primary training hospital is Memorial Hermann with its Level I trauma center. In addition, the Division provides services at LBJ General Hospital and at the M. D. Anderson Cancer Center, where residents rotate through to gain experience in oncological plastic surgery. Residents also do a rotation at St. Joseph's Medical Center, where there are more opportunities to work in cosmetic surgery, as compared to Memorial Hermann, where they are more oriented to trauma and reconstructive surgery. Residents gain experience with a different group of attending plastic surgeons and in more aesthetic surgery, breast reconstructive surgery, and cleft lip and palate surgery with Dr. Ernest Cronin, the nephew of Dr. Thomas Cronin, mentioned earlier. Parks set up the rotation at St. Joseph's Hospital in the late 1980s with Dr. Thomas Cronin. "And that has been a great experience for our residents and has actually expanded their training milieu," said Parks. "It has offered them this added effort in cosmetic surgery which is obviously pretty popular, these days in particular."[18]

The Division has become known for its expertise in reconstruction: not just burns but also for major trauma reconstruction. But residents gain experience in the whole realm of plastic surgery. Microsurgery has also become a strong suit, with the division developing new techniques and training over fifty surgeons in this subspecialty. "Our microsurgeons have reattached almost everything you can reattach—arms and legs, genitalia, and everything else," said Parks. Among the division's milestones, the development of microsurgery is among the most significant, including its work in the area of anastomosis (a surgical connection between two structures: usually between tubular structures such as blood vessels) of very small vessels under the microscope, with replenishment of the blood supply to tissues. "That involves re-plantation of different parts that have been amputated—fingers, wrists, arms—usually through trauma," said Parks. "That has probably had as great an influence as anything on plastic surgery."

Parks estimated that by 2014, the Division had trained about sixty-five residents in plastic surgery and had produced its share of surgeons who have gone on to have very successful careers. "Our current craniofacial surgeon, Dr. John Teichgraeber, trained with us here, and he stayed with the program," said Parks. Dr. Robert McCauley went on to become Chief Plastic Surgeon at the Shriners Burns Institute in Galveston. Three former residents, Drs. Peter Ledoux, Oscar Ochoa, and Steve Pisano, are now together in San Antonio and manage one of the most advanced and renowned breast reconstructive services in the country. Dr. Mimi Leong is now the Chief of Plastic Surgery at the VA Hospital in Houston, and Drs. Scott Oats and Gregg Reis are now professors at M. D. Anderson Cancer Center.[19]

Advances in acute care and all of its components have been among the hallmarks of the Department of Surgery throughout its history. Its surgical specialists in all the related areas have continued to conduct research, provide exceptional patient care, and train new generations of surgeons.

But there is more to the Department of Surgery than its acute care group. In 2014, twenty years after Richard Andrassy first stepped in to help out on an interim basis, the Department of Surgery included seven specialty divisions: Acute Care Surgery, Elective General Surgery, General Surgery/LBJ, Immunology and Organ Transplantation, Oral and Maxillofacial Surgery, Plastic and Reconstructive Surgery, and Urology. Over the years, what was once known simply as General Surgery and the Division of Urology have remained two of the mainstays of the department, creating newer and better options for patients, and training a new generation in what might be described as classical surgery. But new developments in these areas, along with the passing of time and changing of the guard in terms of divisional leadership, presented new opportunities and some unique challenges for the department and its chairman, Richard Andrassy. Staffed with highly motivated, dedicated faculty, the department would continue to meet new challenges and explore the new frontiers of surgery, thereby fulfilling its mission of teaching, research, and patient care in ways most people could never imagine.

CHAPTER 8

Evolution of the Department

General Surgery, Urology, and Immunology and Organ Transplantation

Another significant factor in the evolution of the Department of Surgery over the years had actually occurred near the end of Frank Moody's tenure as chairman. This was the opening of the Harris County Hospital District's new Lyndon Baines Johnson General Hospital (LBJ) on June 2, 1989, and the subsequent affiliation agreement between the hospital district and the medical school signed in January 1990. Although the addition of a new teaching hospital provided wider opportunities and more cases for medical students and residents, it also brought new responsibilities for the school's academic departments, including surgery. "It started off out there in [July] 1990," recalled Dr. Richard Andrassy. "It was basically just a small county hospital with Dr. Ron Fischer, who was Chief of Surgery. There were only a handful of us out there at the time, one or two other guys and me. I would go out and do general and pediatric surgery."

When it first opened, the hospital offered a limited range of surgical services, but during its first decade it quickly developed an increasing demand in both general and pediatric surgery. This in turn added to the administrative load while providing a developmental arena for new faculty to gain experience, potentially as a proving ground for future division heads or chiefs. Andrassy noted that occasionally when he hired new faculty he would assign them to LBJ to give them the experience of handling the pressure of running a busy service. After Ron Fischer, Dr. John Potts served as Chief of Surgery and gained valuable administrative experience that he later put to good use as the Department of Surgery's Program Director. Then in 1998, Andrassy appointed Dr. David Mercer

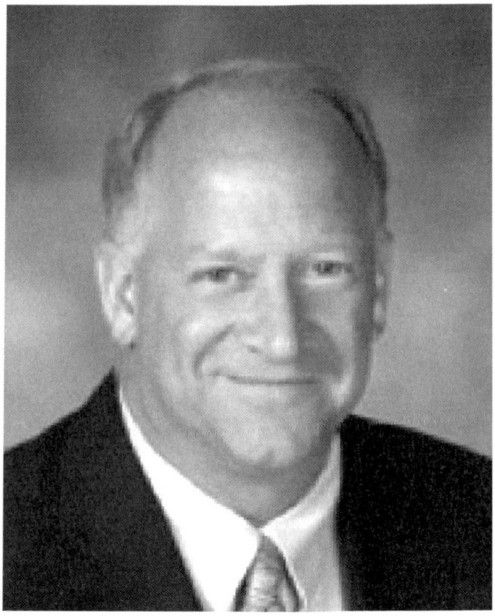

David Mercer, MD.

to serve as Chief of Surgery. Mercer was a national leader in surgery and elected president of the prestigious Society of University Surgeons. At LBJ Hospital, Mercer, too, learned the ropes of running an increasingly busy service and served as chief for about eight years. By 2006, he was ready for a change and stepped down from this position to concentrate on his teaching and administrative roles as Division Director of General Surgery at UT and Chief of General Surgery at Hermann Hospital. In 2009, he was appointed Chairman of the Department of Surgery at the University of Nebraska Medical Center.[1]

Meanwhile, through Dr. Mercer and others, Richard Andrassy had become acquainted with Dr. Tien C. Ko, a young associate professor of surgery, biochemistry, and molecular biology who was teaching at UTMB in Galveston. At the time Ko had a grant from the National Institutes of Health (NIH) with which he was running a laboratory and conducting research. He also was president of the Association of Academic Surgeons. Ko later acknowledged that although he enjoyed doing research, he also wanted to be more involved in mentoring young surgeons. When Andrassy approached him about possibly making the move to Houston, Dr. Ko was intrigued at the prospect. "This opportunity came along to become Chief of Surgery at the county hospital," said Ko.

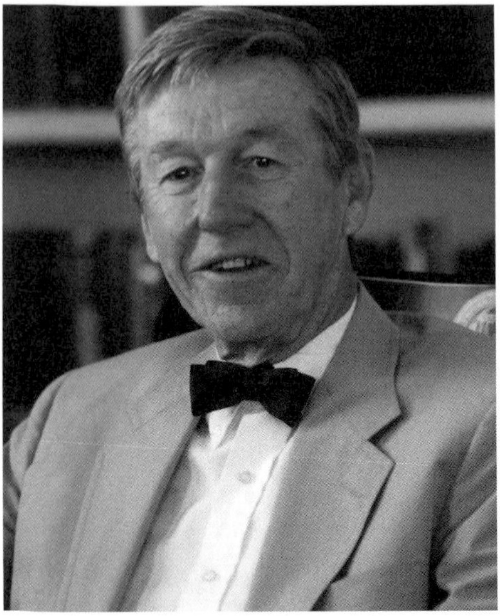

Cheves M. Smythe, MD. Smythe served twice as dean of the Medical School, 1970-75 and as interim dean, 1995-96.

"I thought it was perfect timing for me to transition from just having my own practice and research to move into more of a leadership role." On February 1, 2007, Dr Tien C. Ko formally took over as Chief of Surgery at Lyndon B. Johnson General Hospital and Professor of Surgery at the Medical School.[2]

Initially, as Ko settled in at LBJ, he found a surgical service set in an environment in which the institutional culture was at odds with the vision of the Medical School. Because its initial mission was to provide obstetrics services, the hospital struggled to find its identity during the months after it first opened. When it became a UT affiliate in 1990, the mission changed to that of a general medical and surgical hospital, a function of which its soon-to-be Chief of Medical Service and former dean of the Medical School, Cheves M. Smythe wryly observed, "was not the function for which it was designed or built." Smythe later noted that much of the old Jefferson Davis Hospital staff had transferred to LBJ, bringing the values and attitudes of the old hospital along with them. Davis had been a public hospital relegated to providing a chest service for chronic tuberculosis patients and obstetrics services before it was closed. This type of patient care was much different from what would be expected from the staff in an acute-care general hospital. Smythe noted that when he assumed his post leading the LBJ Hospital medical service in 1991, "it was immediately apparent that the nursing service and the professional staff were in different worlds, did not know each other, had only the most haphazard of interchanges. Although not overtly hostile, there was no sense of working together as a functioning team." Nevertheless, Smythe saw in LBJ a wonderful opportunity on which to build, a place brimming with potential. But it would take a long while to reinvent the institutional culture, a culture that would inevitably impact the surgery service.[3]

Tien Ko, then, began recruiting staff in surgical specialties badly needed at LBJ, particularly in minimally invasive surgery and surgical oncology. For faculty, he brought in surgeons who were fellowship-trained and also possessed a strong desire to teach. Because of their expanded range of expertise, his new hires had an almost immediate impact on the residents. Now, instead of just doing basic hernia and gallbladder surgery, residents occasionally had opportunities to work a few major cases. And for Ko, the addition of new faculty brought him credibility as chief and signaled the beginning of a new era in the department. Still, it took time for the culture to change, but new residents coming in quickly bought into a program that now emphasized greater cooperation among surgeons, nurses, and anesthesiologists--all key people in bringing efficiency to the operating room and improving the patients' experience and outcomes. Although LBJ had only nine operating rooms at the time, the volume of cases soon doubled, and the team began to consider how to expand further. "I like to think a lot of it had to do with our quality," said Ko. "We got more involved in being more efficient in the OR." The steadily increasing volume and the improving efficiency inspired confidence in Ko's leadership, and soon he was able to convince the hospital district's administrators to support using the operating rooms on a seven-day-a-week, around-the-clock basis. Ko reasoned that with some 45 percent of the surgical volume coming from the emergency room during the daytime, if he could convince faculty on duty at night to operate during those hours, they could schedule elective surgeries like gallbladders without having to cancel them due to the number of emergency surgery cases that arrived during the day.[4]

During the next few years, several changes at the hospital, including

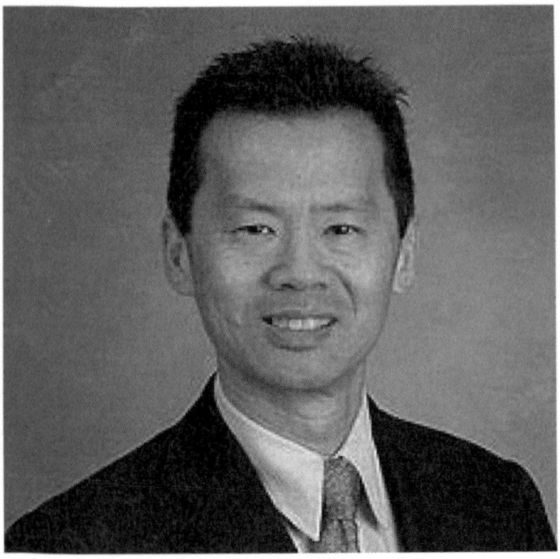

Tien C. Ko, MD.

construction of a new outpatient facility, also served to improve the surgical service. When Ko first arrived, LBJ had nine operating rooms, but three of them were very small. The hospital district agreed to a redesign and converted the three small operating rooms into two larger rooms that were more efficient but that also reduced the total to eight ORs. The increase in minimally invasive surgery led to the addition of updated laparoscopic equipment and more ceiling-mounted equipment, which in turn removed floor clutter and the necessity of moving things around in the operating rooms, which further improved conditions. Still, there was an obvious need for more ORs. As a response to the hospital's growing patient load, in October 2013, a new, three-story outpatient center opened adjacent to the original hospital building, increasing clinic space by about 30 percent. During the spring of 2014, five new operating rooms opened on the third floor, yielding a total of thirteen now state-of-the-art, operating rooms. The five new operating rooms would handle ambulatory cases and elective surgery, which meant expanded services for the community and a broader experience for the surgical residents. LBJ General Hospital could now offer a wide variety of surgical care for patients including general surgery, surgical oncology, head and neck surgery, urology, plastic surgery, GYN surgery, oral and maxillofacial surgery, and eye surgery—basically every type of surgery except cardiac, bypass, spinal, neurosurgery, and burn surgery.[5]

In addition, LBJ has a bustling emergency room, and with 70,000 emergency patient visits annually, it is one of the busiest Level III Trauma Centers in the nation. It is important to note that while Harris Health System operates sixteen community centers, there are only two county hospitals in Harris County: Ben Taub, located in the Texas Medical Center, and LBJ, situated northeast of downtown. Ben Taub has a certified Level I Trauma Center and, along with the nearby Level I Trauma Center at Memorial Hermann Hospital, generally stays busy with severe trauma cases. This means that during extremely busy periods at Ben Taub, less critical emergency patients generally are redirected to LBJ for care. At LBJ, the trauma surgeons are all certified by the American College of Surgeons in Advanced Trauma Life Support (ATLS), and a trauma surgeon is on duty twenty-fours a day to take care of emergency cases.[6]

By 2014, Lyndon B. Johnson General Hospital had matured into an acute care facility with 328 licensed beds, offering a full range of medical services. It also had a key role as one of the Medical School's major teaching hospitals. "LBJ is the most important gift to this medical school for all the residency training and the students because of the unbelievable [variety in] types of patients we see," said Ko. Demographics show that the hospital serves patients who generally are from lower socioeconomic levels and who often are either underinsured or completely lacking health insurance. "Because we are a county facility and many of them do not have primary care doctors, or they have poor access to healthcare, many of the patients present with diseases that are very advanced," said Ko. "We also see very unique diseases, infectious disease from South America, and things that you may not see in a suburban hospital. That presents a lot of opportunity for our residents and students to learn. So, yes, the patients, their great attitude, and the pathology that they bring in—[the experience] is incredible."[7]

UT's residents generally find their rotations at LBJ to be very rewarding, in part because they have an opportunity to do a lot of "doctoring" on real patients. Dr. Eduardo Souchon, who has been on staff and teaching at LBJ hospital since July 2003, noted that being at LBJ is rewarding for the full-time surgical staff as well as for the residents. "It is a really fantastic experience for me," stated Souchon. "And in my [medical] practice life, teaching and being here has been very rewarding. I think LBJ is probably the best teaching institution in the state, because the residents are

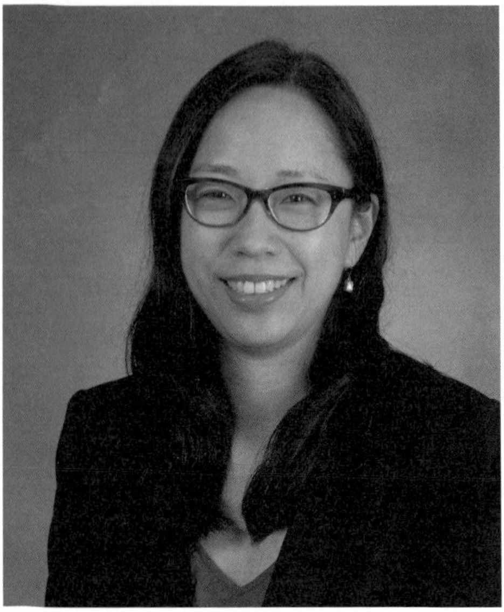

Lillian S. Kao, MD.

doing things that they would not be able to do at other places." Because there are no surgery fellows at LBJ, the residents are at the top of the hierarchy and therefore have the opportunity to take significant responsibility in caring for the patients. They see a broader range of pathology and, if they get a difficult case, they have to take care of that patient. "They understand that the patients are really grateful and that they are providing a service to the community," Ko observed. "There is a really unique, vulnerable population of patients that you do not see anywhere else. And then, the people that work here—whether nurses or administrators or physicians—they are very committed to the hospital and to the patients. And that is what makes it so special—people are here really by choice. It is a great group to work with." The affiliation agreement between The University of Texas Health Science Center at Houston (UT Health) and the Harris County Hospital District (now known as Harris Health) has been fruitful for both institutions. LBJ Hospital has the benefit of having the medical school's highly experienced medical faculty and talented young residents providing clinical services for its patients. And for the medical school and its department of surgery, the affiliation broadens the range of responsibilities and provided new opportunities for both surgical faculty and residents.[8]

The addition of the new Division of General Surgery/LBJ and its subsequent expansion was undoubtedly a major milestone in the history of the department. A second historical turning point that ultimately had a great impact on the department actually began during the late 1980s with the development of new technology that fundamentally changed the nature of general surgery and led to the evolving new field of minimally invasive surgery. Dr. Bruce V. MacFadyen Jr. had played a key role in the department from the beginning, first as Senior Resident and then as faculty, working in concert with Drs. Dudrick, Duke, and Copeland, to establish the department during the 1970s. Early in his career, he became interested in flexible endoscopy and by the 1980s saw the developing trend toward less invasive surgery as having a significant role in the future. "We thought it was going to be the flexible endoscope, because at that time, there had been the development of biliary endoscopy called ERCP [Endoscopic Retrograde Cholangiopancreatography]," said MacFadyen. Frank Moody, department chair at the time, supported MacFadyen's request to take some additional training in flexible endoscopy. In 1986, MacFadyen spent three months in Cleveland, Ohio, with Dr. Jeffrey Ponsky, a surgeon at Mount Sinai Hospital, who had developed a technique called Percutaneous Endoscopic Gastrostomy [PEG] whereby a surgeon placed feeding tubes into the stomach with a flexible endoscope.[9] MacFadyen learned the technique working with Ponsky, and then they began to expand its application. "I got in on the ground floor with that, and I got a whole new and expanded appreciation of where flexible endoscopy was going," said MacFadyen. "I brought that technique back here and we started doing endoscopy." MacFadyen continued to develop his skills and took additional ERCP training with experts in Canada. He worked with radiologists at the medical school to develop a new technique in which they were able to access the gallbladder percutaneously (through a needle-puncture of the skin instead of by opening the skin with a scalpel) and remove stones from the gallbladder. MacFadyen collected data on the procedure and presented a paper at a then fairly small laparoscopic flexible endoscopy surgical group, the Society of American Gastrointestinal and Endoscopic Surgeons (SAGES), in 1988.[10]

Following the presentation, he met a French surgeon at the conference who told him about a new technique they were using in France:

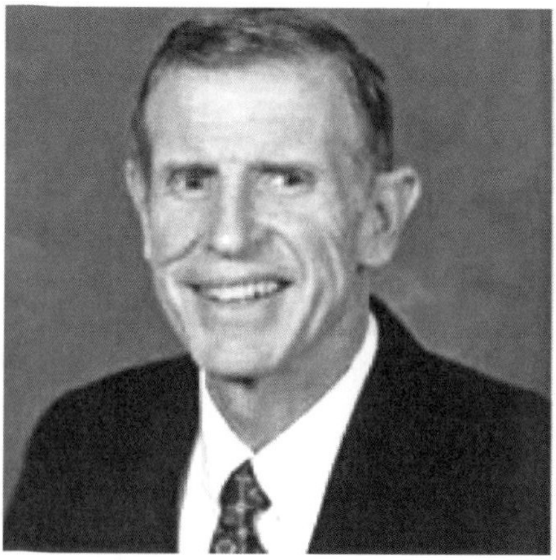

Bruce V. MacFadyen, Jr., MD.

laparoscopic cholecystectomy (removal of the gall bladder). "I looked at that and I realized that is where the action was for surgery rather than this percutaneous procedure," MacFadyen recalled years later. He went to Utah to learn the technique, so new that even the surgeons who served as instructors had performed only a few of the procedures. "It was almost the blind leading the blind, but we learned this thing," said MacFadyen. "I came back here, we got some equipment together, and we started doing our first case—I think in 1989. And everything is history from there as far as the development of laparoscopic cholecystectomy and then laparoscopic everything, which we are doing now. That is how it got started." MacFadyen credits Frank Moody with having the foresight to see the significance of the new procedures and with encouraging him to pursue his interest in the new field. The laparoscopic surgery practice began to grow, and soon UT surgeons were doing inguinal hernias, then ventral hernias, colon resections, spleens, and finding other applications. Although today surgeons sometimes still utilize the more invasive technique for very severe cases, minimally invasive surgery has become the preferred option for more surgeons and patients. The smaller incision means quicker recovery, reduced risk of infections, and, as a side benefit, is less obvious cosmetically. Patients can go home earlier, and today, even cholecystectomies often are done as an outpatient procedure. "We developed our own practice here and it really grew," said MacFadyen. "We were one of the first groups to start that sort of thing. So, yes, those are some of the first things that were done here."[11]

This soon led to the department working closely with manufacturers including US Surgical (now known as Covidien) and Ethicon Endo-surgery (now known as Ethicon, a division of Johnson & Johnson) to develop new instruments and equipment. MacFadyen found the work challenging and enjoyable. He recalled that in the early days, it might take about eighteen months to go from concept to the actual availability of a new instrument. But eventually, improvement of the development process made it possible to design a new product and go to production in a shorter period of time, sometimes in the range of three to five months. MacFadyen noted that companies like Ethicon and US Surgical wanted to be in the forefront of new technology and through the years have worked closely with surgeons. "When I needed an instrument to do a particular task, they would develop it," said MacFadyen. "It was just a fun time, because they were responsive to the changes." One area of concern related to the ergonomics of the instruments themselves. It became a serious problem if a surgeon was working for long periods, three to four hours or more, because the pressure of the instrument against nerves in their hand often led to numbness. The surgical supply companies became sensitive to that and responded with modifications to their equipment in order to allow longer surgeries without causing numbness in the hand or fingers.[12] Over time, the laparoscope became the mainstay for much of general surgery. In addition, the flexible endoscope has evolved with improved optics, light transmission, and high definition. The newer instruments are vastly improved compared to those early days, and this has led to innovative and improved surgical techniques too.[13]

MacFadyen continued to teach and practice surgery at the Medical School throughout the 1990s. In 2002, an opportunity arose for him to become Chairman of Surgery at Georgia Regents University in Augusta, Georgia. He decided to accept the appointment beginning April 1, 2002. His departure left Richard Andrassy short handed in the area of laparoscopic surgery. But, in the spring of 2002, Dr. Erik B. Wilson was just completing a Laparoendoscopic Fellowship with Philip L. Leggett, MD, one of the pioneers of laparoscopy in Houston. Wilson, who was born and raised in the small town of Andrews, in West Texas, anticipated developing his own surgical practice in a rural town, but decided first to see what opportunities might arise in the Houston area. Dr. David Mercer, who was Chief of Surgery at LBJ Hospital at that time, had heard about Wilson and encouraged Andrassy to consider offering him a position at the Medical School. With MacFadyen leaving for Georgia, there were no laparoscopic people in the department, and Andrassy wanted to maintain some balance on the faculty between trauma and elective general surgery. After interviewing Wilson, Andrassy offered him a position at UT. "I did not think I was going to be in academics, and I never thought I would come back to the Medical Center, even though I did my medical school training here [Baylor College of Medicine]," Wilson recalled years later. "I grew up in a small town, so I did not think I would ever be a big city guy. But I decided I'd take the job and see what happens."[14]

In addition to Wilson, Andrassy also hired Dr. Terry Scarborough, who had done his surgical residency and fellowship training in laparoscopic surgery at Baylor College of Medicine as well, and Dr. Steven Glorsky, a trauma surgeon who had become interested in weight loss surgery.[15] Glorsky worked with Frank Moody in the Bariatric Surgical Center for a time and then left UT to go into private practice. Meanwhile, Wilson anticipated that he and Scarborough, as advanced laparoscopic surgeons, would be doing surgery for hernias, gallbladders, colons, and solid organs, but at the time Bariatric Surgery was coming more into its own. Wilson found that laparoscopic referrals had dropped off, and in order to increase the volume of patients, he and Scarborough began doing more weight-loss surgery. "We started over from scratch, and the way to get busy was to go straight to the patients," said Wilson. "We started talking about weight-loss surgery and we started doing it. We got into it because it was very technically challenging: operating on morbidly obese patients, helping them lose weight." He found doing the procedures to be extremely rewarding, because the patients were so grateful about their outcomes, likening their experience to a kind of "rebirth" after their surgery.[16]

Wilson noted that at the time, there was some bias against obesity treatment, and Bariatric Surgery was viewed by many in the general surgery community as being out of the mainstream. "If you were doing it,

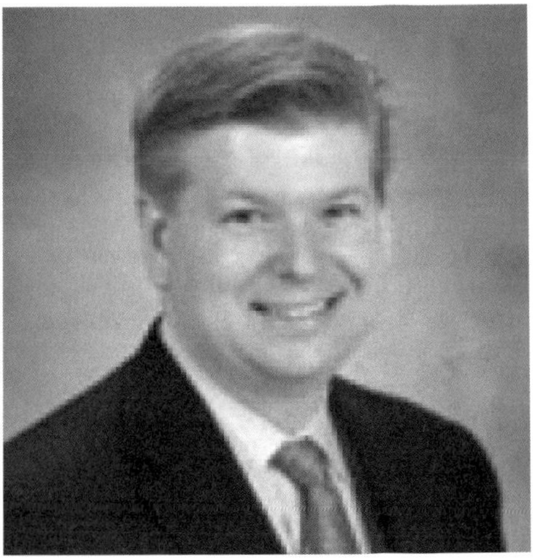

Erik B. Wilson, MD.

some people thought you might be kind of a hack," Wilson recalled. "So we had a lot to overcome. They did not really want us to have our clinic down in the Medical Center, so they put us in an outside clinic out at the West Loop near the Galleria, because that clinic was not very busy." Wilson and Scarborough soon noticed that they were attracting a large volume of patients, and their outpost clinic began making a handsome profit. The patients liked the free parking, and they did not have to deal with finding their way in the sprawling Texas Medical Center. As time passed, it became obvious to Wilson and Scarborough that they had enough business to build their own satellite clinic. They found a suitable location outside the Texas Medical Center, in nearby Bellaire, Texas, and the UT Specialty Surgery Center was born. Subsequently, it has grown into something of a "west campus" for the medical school. Now UT offers a wide range of services at the clinic, including family practice and specialists in dermatology, gynecology, and gastroenterology. Wilson explained that the basic principle behind the patient attraction to minimally invasive surgery is that if patients have a choice and the outcomes are the same as far as results and safety, then patients would prefer an operation that was done through a less invasive approach. Regarding the success of their surgical service, he observed: "It made us focus on acting like a private practice. I wanted to create a culture where we have a very patient-friendly environment. Our business is set up around making sure patients are happy and that they choose us, because they can choose any surgeon to do their operation. It is not an emergency [procedure]."[17]

As Wilson and Scarborough continued to develop their surgical practice, they also considered the notion of creating a fellowship to train other surgeons in laparoscopic minimally invasive surgery. Wilson established a fellowship program in 2003 and began training two fellows per year in the one-year fellowship program. "We also felt it would be interesting to extend the experience of the fellows, so we created what we called the Fellowship Consortium," said Wilson. He saw that some of the other laparoscopic surgeons in Houston, Drs. Phillip Leggett and Patrick Reardon, had fellows, and he knew of an active laparoscopic surgical group in San Antonio. As he recalled later: "We decided, why not create a process or an infrastructure where everyone could work together? We created a consortium, and although these fellowships were technically independent; we ended up putting them all [together] through UT so they could have good benefits and be protected under the UT umbrella." The result was the Minimally Invasive Fellowship Consortium which is part of Minimally Invasive Surgeons of Texas (MIST). "Minimally Invasive Surgeons of Texas is basically a brand that I wanted to come up with to get people to understand that we are a different type of surgeon," said Wilson. "We are focused on doing surgery through scopes or through the most minimally invasive process that we can. A minimally invasive surgeon is a weird specialty, in that you are not a specialty of an organ system or a disease state or anything like that; you are basically a specialist of technology."[18]

The new fellowship program was innovative on several levels. Fellows would work in both private and academic environments, rotating between minimally invasive surgical practices in Houston and in San Antonio. The idea behind this was to expand the fellowship experience and make it attractive to good candidates. The University of Texas Minimally Invasive Surgery Fellowship offers advanced training in laparoscopic, endoscopic, and minimally invasive surgery. By taking advantage of the opportunity to rotate between busy practices in San Antonio and Houston, fellows gain broad experience in all phases of laparoscopic surgery including bariatrics, Nissen fundoplication, laparoscopic donor nephrectomy, laparoscopic colectomy, laparoscopic hernia repair, and flexible endoscopy. Dr. Eric Haas, a graduate of the Medical School, is the founder and president of Colorectal Surgical Associates (CSA) in Houston. Haas serves as Program Director of the Minimally Invasive Colon and Rectal Surgery Fellowship Program at the Medical School. CSA provides opportunities for fellows to gain experience using minimally invasive techniques to diagnose and treat colon and rectal problems, colon cancer, and colorectal surgery with flexible endoscopes. In addition, Drs. Patrick Reardon and Brian Dunkin provide a high volume of advanced laparoscopic surgical experience where fellows work with advanced flexible endoscopes, endoscopic retrograde cholangiopancreatography (ERCP), natural orifice translumenal endoscopic surgery (NOTES), and advanced general laparoscopic surgery with complex foregut surgeries. Wilson's mentor in laparoscopy, Dr. Phillip L. Leggett, is also part of the fellowship consortium.[19]

Since it was first established in 2003, the MIST Consortium has become one of the largest minimally invasive fellowship programs in the country and trains from six to eight fellows per year, with over fifty trained in its short history. During the years since Wilson first arrived

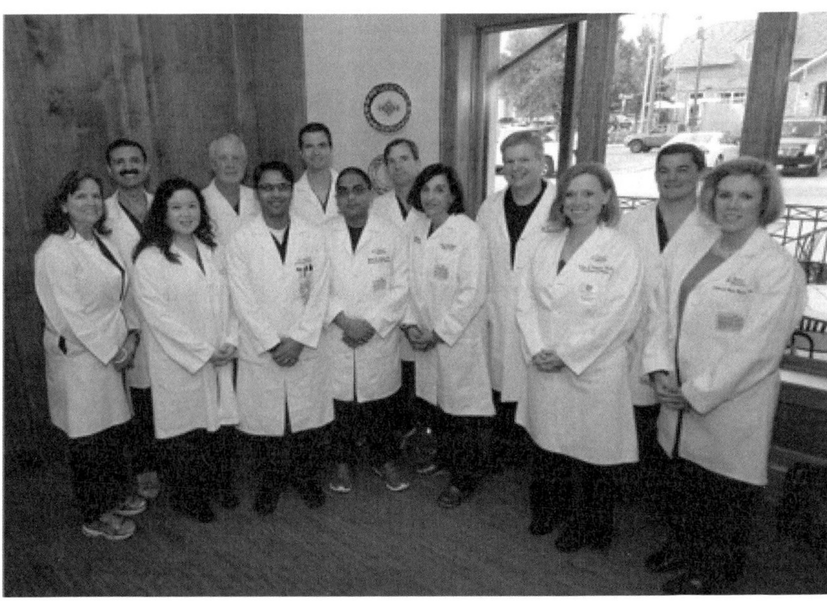

Minimally Invasive Surgeons of Texas (MIST).

at UT, medical students and residents have become more intrigued and interested in learning how to perform minimally invasive surgery. Wilson recalled, however, that when he first launched the fellowship program he had to work hard at recruiting residents for the MIST fellowships, because they thought it was unnecessary fellowship training, something that should be a part of general surgery. "When I first got here ... I got laughed out of the room a lot when I suggested doing some of it [surgery] laparoscopically," he recalled. But now that the procedure has become commonplace, those views changed and today, many of the MIST fellows come from the ranks of UT residents. The fellows interact together and attend monthly educational meetings and journal clubs. There also is a Morbidity and Mortality Conference that both fellows and residents on the service attend together. As the Division has continued to grow, the fellowships have played a major role in bringing new surgeons on board as faculty. With ten surgeons in the Division of Elective General Surgery by 2014, six were minimally invasive and bariatric, and four of that group came from the MIST fellowship. "We trained them and then they stayed with us," said Wilson. "We are continuing to do that today, and it has allowed us to really grow our group. And, that is how the Minimally Invasive Fellowship Consortium developed."[20]

In addition to developing a large minimally invasive surgery practice, the Division of Elective General Surgery has taken a leading role in Robotic Surgery. Initially, the first robotic platform came as a result of UT recruiting Dr. Hazim Safi to become Chairman of Cardiothoracic and Vascular Surgery when it became a separate department in 1999. Many thought robotic surgery would become a major component of heart surgery, but the robot was not utilized as much as first expected. "We started playing around with surgical robotics at that time, and I started using them for bariatric cases early on," said Wilson. "It continued to grow and develop, and now we are doing 400–500 cases a year with the robot. We have been doing it for over ten years and we are one of the big houses in the world as far as general surgeons that use the robot." Robotics is used increasingly in urology, gynecology, and now in general surgery. Advantages of the robot are that it augments the surgeon's visualization and provides extra dexterity, because the instruments match the movement of the fingers and wrists, allowing for greater surgical preci-

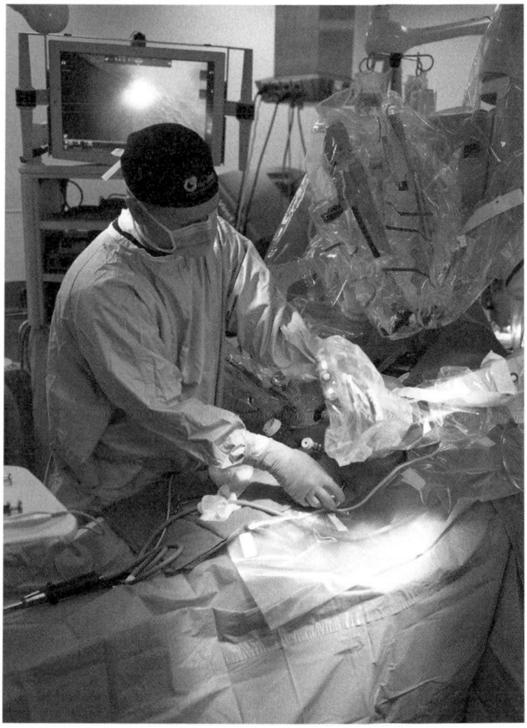

Dr. Erik Wilson preparing a patient and robot for surgery.

sion. These new procedures include nearly every bariatric operation, hernia repairs, reflux surgery, and more recently, complex revisional cases. Patients who have had previous bariatric surgery somewhere else in the country now come to MIST at UT for help with problems or complications. "Our practice has evolved [to] where we went from primary bariatric surgeons to doing lots of revisional cases," Wilson explained. "In revisional cases when you have been in the abdomen a couple of times, it gets very dense and scarred, and re-dissecting everything out can be difficult. But with robotics we can do very complicated revisional cases safely."[21]

Elective General Surgery also has become focused on endoluminal surgery, which is surgery performed through endoscopes generally inserted through the mouth but sometimes through the rectum. During the past four or five years, several endoluminal devices and platforms have been developed for use in reflux and weight-loss surgery, other stomach procedures, and even a few colon procedures. Surgeons now are able to go from inside the mouth to the stomach to perform weight-loss surgery,

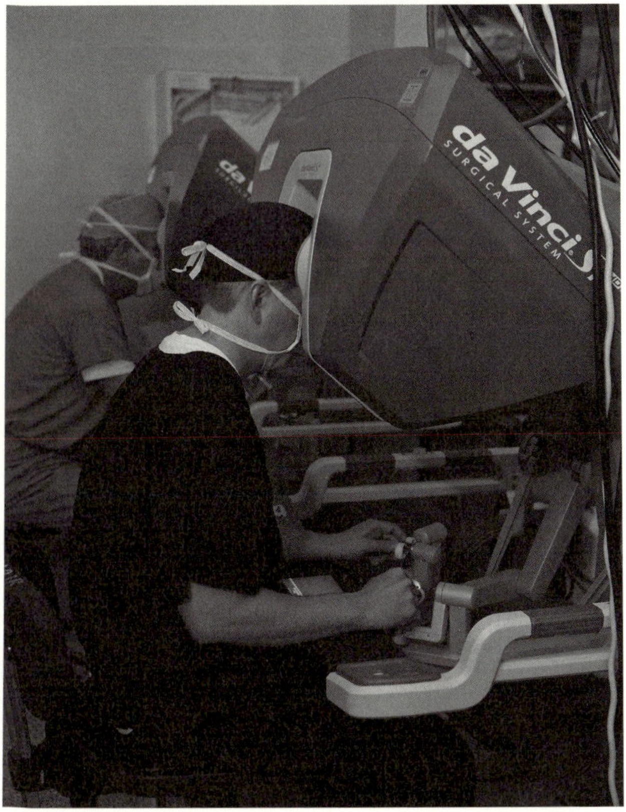

Dr. Erik Wilson training a fellow in robotic surgery.

or from the rectum up to the colon. "We are doing several studies on transoral weight loss surgery, transoral anti-reflux surgery, and transoral resection of tumors," said Wilson. "We think that has a huge future, because it does not have any incisions, so patients are very interested in it because there is no incision on the belly at all." These new procedures hold great promise, and when combined with robotics, new digital platforms will enable surgeons to perform very precise, complex surgery inside the stomach through the patient's mouth without making incisions or making only very strategic, small incisions in certain areas where scars would remain unseen—virtually scarless surgery.[22]

This growing expertise in robotic surgery has led to both greater demand and to international renown. By 2014, the division had three robots in the operating room and five in the training lab. They have trained some 1,000 surgical teams over the past ten years, many of whom came from all over the world to learn robotics. They also have trained surgical teams for hernia repairs and in advanced laparoscopic and advanced flexible endoscopy. Wilson observed that the robotic training center is very little known outside the surgical community and is not well advertised. But he allows that while other institutions now do their own robotic training, for a time almost everyone in the Texas Medical Center who had received training in robotics received their training at UT, "because we were the first and longest standing robotics training center in the South." In addition to training surgical teams in robotics, UT surgeons also have worked with manufacturers in developing new products and procedures. Among the firms are Intuitive Surgical, which makes the Da Vinci Robot, and a number of endoluminal companies. "Basically our skill set has been in procedure development," said Wilson. "We grew that out of our robotics lab, because we had that training center from the very beginning. We have continued to work on using that training center to grow and develop new procedures, and we do it on endoluminal platforms as well as robotic platforms."[23]

Looking back, Wilson noted several key milestones that enabled the division to develop. First, he credits Rich Andrassy for making the decision to hire a group focused on minimally invasive and elective surgery, which allowed the department to expand its capabilities. Next was the decision to create the fellowship program, which added a new educational component, followed by the work with robotics and creating new, innovative techniques. Within a short time, Wilson noted that they began building their division "from the inside." As he observed, "We had really good trainees and they ended up being very good surgeons." This led to hiring minimally invasive surgery specialists Dr. Brad Snyder (UT Health Fellowship, Minimally Invasive Surgery and Elective General Surgery 2007–2008) and Dr. Todd Wilson (UT Health Fellowship, Minimally Invasive and Elective General Surgery Fellowship 2008–2009). "We started growing very quickly, and now we are truly a comprehensive elective general surgery division."[24]

The success of the minimally invasive surgery program was one factor that soon led Andrassy to create a new organizational structure within the department, and the Division of Elective General Surgery was born. As Wilson recalled, "Over time, I had evolved into being the chief of a division that really did not exist to what now is an actual division [in the department]." The practice has expanded from its primary focus on Bar-

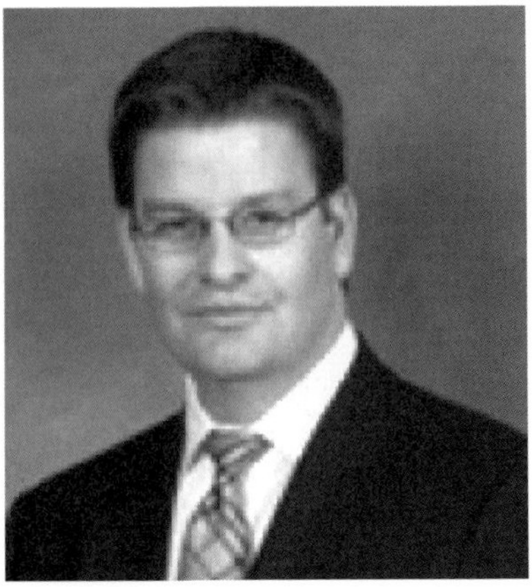

Donald P. Lesslie, III, DO.

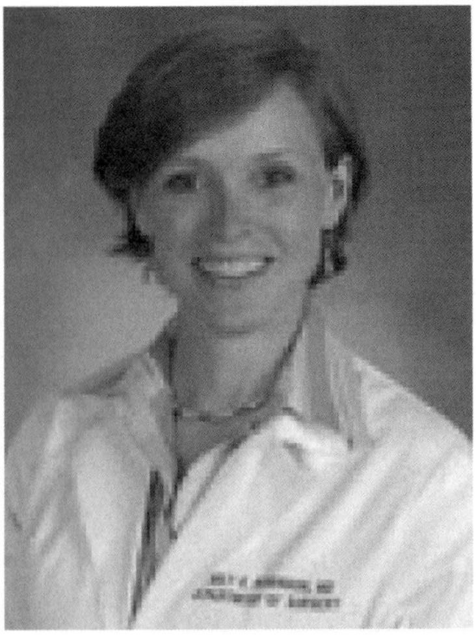

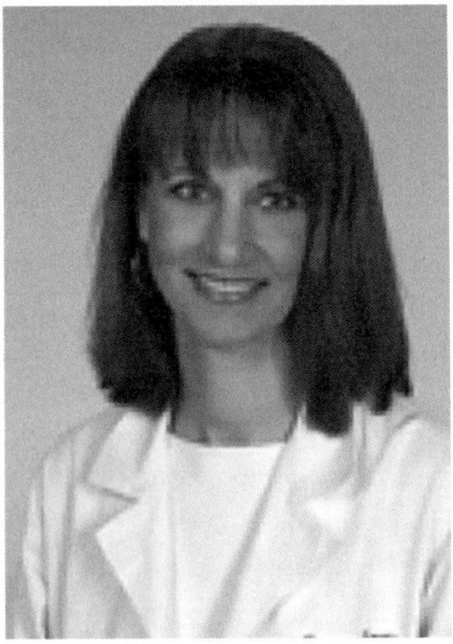

Left to right: Emily Robinson, MD. Rosemary Kozar, MD.

iatric Surgery to a wide range of elective surgery. The division has two surgical oncologists, Donald P. Lesslie, MD, and Rebecca L. Wiatrek, MD, who do advanced cancer surgery including pancreas, stomach, liver, and more complex procedures. Emily Robinson, MD, does breast surgery and endocrinology. In addition to surgical oncology and bariatrics, the division also provides foregut surgery for reflux, complex abdominal wall reconstruction, hernia repairs, colorectal surgery, and general surgery. By 2014, the Division of Elective General Surgery and the MIST Fellowship Consortium had become well known nationally for having a very strong fellowship program and for its large bariatric practice. Internationally, the Division is known for robotics and now, with a major role in FDA trials with endoluminal therapies, the division is gaining renown for endoluminal expertise as well. Today, the division has grown into a broad, elective general surgery practice.[25]

While Elective General Surgery was evolving over time, so too was the Division of Urology, one of the oldest components of the Department of Surgery. In 1974, Department Chair Stan Dudrick successfully recruited his former colleague at the University of Pennsylvania, Joseph N. Corriere Jr., MD to be the director of the Division of Urology. Corriere, whose father was an urologist, received his MD at Seton Hall College of Medicine, did his internship at the Pennsylvania Hospital in Philadelphia, and continued postgraduate training at the University of Pennsylvania. Upon arriving in Houston, he found himself part of a department with only three or four people in General Surgery and that he was director of a surgical division with one surgeon—himself. He saw that in addition to teaching and developing a clinical practice, he needed to recruit faculty and residents to build the division. Many of Corriere's early faculty recruits and residents became renowned for the expertise they developed in their subspecialties and frequently accepted prestigious positions at other institutions, further enhancing the reputation of the Medical School. Among his first faculty recruits was Larry I. Lipschultz, MD, who had worked with Corriere during his residency at the University of Pennsylvania and specialized in infertility and sexual dysfunction. Lipschultz came to the Medical School on a two-year fellowship in male reproductive medicine, started his own lab, and soon developed a large practice in male infertility. "Larry quickly rose to being a full professor, published papers, got grants, did research, did all the right things," said Corriere. After two years at The University of Texas, Baylor College of Medicine, which had a much larger reproductive medicine/fertility program, made an offer Lipschultz simply could not turn down. After moving over to Baylor, he continued his work, became a pioneer in urological microsurgery, and achieved recognition as a world-renowned expert in male reproductive medicine. Today, he is Professor of Urology and Chief of the Division of Male Reproductive Medicine and Surgery at the Baylor College of Medicine. "So, that was my first recruit," said Corriere.[26]

Corriere continued to recruit faculty to his division and brought in a young surgeon who also had been a resident at the University of Pennsylvania, George Benson, MD. "George was just a brilliant guy," Corriere recalled. "We had a very good anatomy, uroanatomy department so I got him an American Urological Association (AUA) fellowship to come and spend two years with the uroanatomy group here. That led to some really great things." One of the things he was able to do was to disprove what had been the long-held belief on how erection occurred in the penis. Benson's research led him to a breakthrough in male erectile dysfunction, pioneering work that helped pave the way for continuing research and the development of erectile dysfunction drugs like Viagra. "That all started with George showing down the line how all this happened," said Corriere. Benson went on to become a full professor, but Corriere remembered him as being more intrigued with academic medicine rather than clinical practice. Eventually, the Food and Drug Administration (FDA) recruited Benson. He had a sterling career and became Deputy Director, Division of Reproductive and Urologic Products.[27]

Although most of the urology residents went on to clinical practice, Corriere recalled two of his residents who later distinguished themselves in academics. Dr. William Steers came to the Medical School from the Medical College of Ohio, in Toledo. Eventually, after completing his residency at UT and making a couple of stops along the way, the University of Virginia recruited him and he became the Chairman of Urology. He also went on to become editor of the *Journal of Urology*, the number-one urology journal in the world. A second resident who went on to a sterling academic career was Dr. Roger R. Dmochowski, who earned his medical degree at UTMB in Galveston. Dmochowski had served in the navy before coming to Houston. He later became nationally known in urology and eventually a full professor in the Department of Urology as well as Director of Female Pelvic Medicine and Reconstructive Urology Fellowship at Vanderbilt University in Nashville, Tennessee.[28]

Early in his own career, while a resident at the University of Pennsylvania, Corriere had gained considerable experience working on kidney transplantation. It was natural then that at the Medical School, the Division of Urology under Corriere's leadership would be deeply involved in the school's organ transplant program as it developed under Barry Kahan

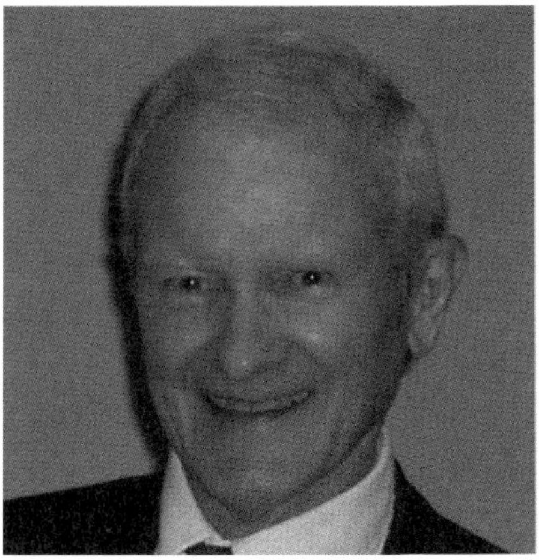

Joseph N. Corriere, Jr., MD.

(see chapter 4). And by the mid-1980s, the urology academic program had developed into a four-year residency in general clinical adult and pediatric urology and in specialized areas including nephrology, histopathology, and metabolic disorders. Residents typically spent about eighteen months under the supervision of the full-time urology staff at Hermann Hospital, six months total in transplant, and six months at M. D. Anderson Hospital learning urologic oncology and also engaged in multidisciplinary training involving general surgery, immunology, urology, and nephrology. Finally, they acquired additional training at the Lithotripsy Unit at St. Joseph's Hospital.[29]

Laboratory research also continued during the 1980s, including the work of Stuart Flechner, who analyzed cell kinetics in cyclosporine-treated kidney recipients; George Benson's work on vascular and neural mechanisms involved in penile erection; and Joseph Corriere's research into reconstructive surgery of the urinary tract and urinary tract trauma. In 1987, the Division of Urology faculty expanded with the arrival of Dr. Jeffery R. Woodside, who had been Professor in the Division of Urology at the University of New Mexico School of Medicine in Albuquerque. During the 1980s and early 1990s, the Division maintained an active clinical practice, developed a new kidney stone center at St. Joseph Hospital, and received accreditation from the AUA to train both residents and practicing urologists in extracorporeal shock wave lithotripsy (ESWL) therapy. ESWL uses shock waves to break up kidney stones into small pieces that can more easily travel through the urinary tract and pass from the body.[30]

In 1992, Jeffrey Woodside announced he was leaving the department to go to into administration at the University of Tennessee at Memphis. Corriere needed to replace him and decided to contact Dr. Edward J. McGuire, Chairman of Urology at the University of Michigan, to see if he had a resident he could recommend to take the place of Woodside. It turned out that McGuire, who was renowned for his work in urodynamics and voiding dysfunction, was looking for a new opportunity. He expressed interest and told Corriere: "I will take the job. I just want you to know I like being chairman." While many division chiefs might have looked askance at McGuire's comment, Corriere later stated that the timing was good for him. He had been division chief since 1974 and also had served for two years as interim chairman of the department. He had recently taken on responsibilities with the AUA and realized that he was ready to relinquish some of his responsibilities within the department. Corriere secured agreements from the department's chair, Frank Moody, and from the dean of the Medical School, John C. Ribble, for McGuire to take over the division once he had settled in. "He was an international figure," Corriere recalled years later. "And, of course, he brought down this huge population of patients. He had the biggest practice in the hospital." After about one year Corriere resigned as Chairman of Urology, remained on the faculty, and continued to work with the AUA.[31]

Corriere had a full professional life during these years and was actively involved in professional associations including leadership roles in the South Central Section of the American Urological Association and the greater American Urological Association. Late in 2001 or early 2002, colleagues from the Urology Department at MD Anderson called to ask for Corriere's help. Cancer patients who were having urological problems needed to see an urologist and could not get appropriate treatment from their cancer specialists. At first, it seemed that if Corriere came to M. D. Anderson for half a day a week, he could run a small clinic that would help the oncologists and provide treatment for the patients. "I went over there and you know, I could have seen patients every day," said Corriere. "They had a large population of patients constantly getting infections in their bladder or kidney stones, not patients with urologic cancers but patients with breast cancer, lung cancer, and other cancers." It quickly became clear that M. D. Anderson had more patients with urological issues than the staff could care for, and Corriere made the decision to leave the Medical School and move across the street on a full-time basis. "That is how I came to be full-time at Anderson, but I was the benign doctor at Anderson. I was not there to take care of cancer," said Corriere. "And by that time, I had been elected the President of the American Urologic Association and that required a lot of traveling. So, it just was a normal sort of progression for me to do that."[32]

Reflecting on the changes in Urology since he first began to practice, Corriere noted the decrease in actual surgery and the increase in medical therapy. New drugs, including Proscar and alpha blockers, were developed with the result that many benign conditions formerly treated with surgery are now treated medically. And new technology, including the development of the lithotripter, has really changed open urology. "I think we have decreased open urology something like 60 percent from what we used to do," Corriere observed. Advances in the treatment of cancer, particularly Wilm's Tumors in children and testicular cancer, have been almost miraculous with effective chemotherapy. Wilm's tumors, when diagnosed in a child, now have over a 90 percent cure rate. In testicular tumors, if the tumor is limited to the testicle, the cure rate is over 90 percent, and metastasis to the lungs has a 70 percent cure rate. As Corriere prepared to step away from the Medical School, advances in urology also mirrored what was happening in some of the other surgical specialties.[33]

After six years at UT, in 1999 Ed McGuire decided to return to Michigan. Faculty came and went over the years, leaving Rich Andrassy to fill in occasionally as Division Chief. The Division took a new turn in February 2012 when after a widespread search, Andrassy named Steven E. Canfield, MD, as the new Chief of the Division of Urology. Canfield graduated from Jefferson Medical College at Thomas Jefferson University, in Philadelphia, completed his internship and residency in surgery and urology at Mt. Sinai School of Medicine in New York, and held a three-year fellowship in urologic oncology at MD Anderson Cancer Center. He also acquired further training in robotic assisted radical prostatectomy. Presently Dr. Canfield serves as Chief of Urology at Memorial Hermann–TMC and Lyndon B. Johnson General Hospital as well as Director of the Residency Program in Urology. Canfield is highly regarded both as clinician and educator, receiving numerous honors and awards in his career.[34]

Just months before Canfield's appointment, Andrassy also brought in a new chief for the Division of Immunology and Organ Transplantation, J. Steve Bynon, MD, a nationally recognized leader in abdominal organ transplantation. Dr. Barry Kahan, who as Founding Director had put the Division in the forefront of the organ transplant world, retired as director in 2007. Dr. Charles Van Buren succeeded him as division leader and served for the next four years, until he left to take a position at Baylor College of Medicine in 2011. Since Kahan's arrival in 1976, the transplant surgeons have performed over 3,000 organ transplants at Memorial Hermann Hospital, including the first liver transplant in Houston in 1985. During its history, the division became nationally recognized as one of the leading programs in immunosuppression research and in the use of cyclosporine and rapamycin. In 2011, Bynon's arrival in many ways signaled a new era in organ transplantation at the Medical School and Memorial Hermann-TMC. Bynon came from the University of Alabama at Birmingham, where he had served for eighteen years as director of the liver transplant and pediatric transplant programs. By the time he arrived in Houston, Bynon had performed over 900 liver transplants and had become nationally known for his expertise in pediatric liver and kidney transplantation.[35]

In an era of increasing subspecialization and a continuously expanding array of new technology, The University of Texas Medical School at Houston Department of Surgery has continued to follow the precedent established early on by Stan Dudrick and advanced by his successors, Frank Moody and Richard Andrassy. During the years of Frank Moody's tenure as chair, the notion of what constitutes a traditional department of surgery began to change dramatically, with some of the surgical divisions becoming autonomous departments of their own. This trend continued with his successor, Richard Andrassy, with Pediatric Surgery and Cardiothoracic and Vascular surgery establishing new departments and with Andrassy's visionary restructuring of surgery. In what might have become a period of great turmoil, the steady leadership of Richard Andrassy has instead brought stability to the department and an era of innovation that has placed the department in the forefront of academic surgical programs.

CHAPTER 9

The Shifting Landscape

New Surgical Departments

One of the interesting developments at many medical schools during the past thirty years has been the trend for some of the academic divisions to break away into autonomous, subspecialty departments. There are a number of reasons behind this phenomenon, including the development of sophisticated and expensive new technology, changes in the relations between medical schools and their teaching hospitals, and an improved ability to generate the revenue needed to cover increased costs of compliance with government mandates and to support new research. The development of new technology has fueled these fairly recent organizational changes in a dramatic way, including at the Medical School. "If you start looking at the early 1970s, there was no such thing as ultrasound and CT scan and MRI," said Richard Andrassy. "Everything then was more generalized, and as it has become more technology-driven, you have had to break down into much smaller areas of expertise, because the technology part of it has grown so much." Andrassy recalled that not too many years ago in large academic surgery departments, the faculty was comprised primarily of general surgeons who also had secondary interests in other specific areas. By contrast, today there are more breakaway, specialized surgical departments, in part because surgery has become increasingly "subsubspecialized" as with orthopedic surgeons, for example, who only do knee replacements. The explosion of new technology has also influenced a realignment as specialized surgeons find themselves working more closely with the doctors in their areas, as in pediatric surgeons working with pediatricians, or neurosurgeons working with neurologists. Technology has been the key driving force behind this movement toward subspecialization and in some cases to surgical divisions moving out from under the umbrella of general surgery into autonomous departments. Andrassy noted that some technology, like ultrasound, initially was developed for use in another industry (oil) and then modified for application in medicine. The impact on medicine has been revolutionary. "Hardly any operation I do today is an operation I learned in residency in the early 1970s," said Andrassy. "Every operation—hernia repairs, gallbladders, thyroid surgery—everything is totally different. Appendectomies we do laparoscopically. We used to do them open." New technology and computers have driven this evolution in surgery, and surgeons find that they must evolve too, or they soon will be left behind.[1]

Another sea change in surgery in recent years has been the trend toward medical professionals working together as teams rather than individually. "If you look at the surgeon thirty or forty years ago, it was one individual running the practice, going to the hospital, doing his own thing," observed Andrassy. Today, patients are finding that medicine is adopting more of a team approach to patient care. Thus, one might have a medical doctor, a surgeon, a physical therapist, a nutritionist, and a pharmacist all working as a team in a medical "one-stop-shop" approach. "That is a novel concept for most of the older surgeons, who are used to being independent," said Andrassy. "And now all of a sudden, everything revolves around a team approach to doing things. And that is why I think we have broken away as departments."[2]

Economics is a third driving force behind the changing landscape for medical schools, doctors, and hospitals. "We realized that financially, when you are dealing with a hospital, everything is merging," noted Andrassy. "All practice plans and all doctors have to be affiliated with a big hospital system because, again, it is so technology-driven." Not only medical school departments face these challenges. Private practitioners are finding it increasingly difficult to maintain their offices with the onset of expensive, government-mandated conversions to electronic medical records and a host of new regulations with which they must comply. If they join a larger group, they can share these burdens and also have a stronger negotiating position for better prices with suppliers and managed-care companies.

For these reasons, then, some of the divisions in the Department of Surgery have become autonomous departments over the years. Frank

Moody began to contend with this issue during his term as chairman during the late 1980s regarding Neurosurgery and Orthopaedic Surgery. "Neurosurgery was growing," he recalled years later. "And Orthopaedics ... they wanted to develop their presence at the medical school as full-time orthopedic surgeons. That was a problem that I gradually resolved by making it a department. My first four or five years were spent trying to overcome certain political problems and then get these units established." As discussed previously, by Frank Moody's term as chairman (1982–1994), the Department of Surgery was comprised of several specialized divisions including General Surgery, Immunology and Organ Transplantation, Neurosurgery, Oral and Maxillofacial Surgery, Orthopaedic Surgery, Pediatric Surgery, Plastic and Reconstructive Surgery, Thoracic and Cardiovascular Surgery, and Urology. During the next fifteen years, Neurosurgery, Orthopaedic Surgery, Pediatric Surgery, Otorhinolaryngology–Head and Neck (ENT) Surgery, and Cardiothoracic and Vascular Surgery would also break away to form separate departments. Although it is not the intent of this study to do a full history of these departments, it is important to provide a brief overview here, since they all had their origins in the Department of Surgery. In particular, Pediatric Surgery (covered in chapter 6) and Cardiothoracic and Vascular Surgery have multiple layers of connection to the original department and require a slightly more lengthy treatment.[3]

Neurosurgery

By the mid-1980s, the Division of Neurosurgery was thriving within the department and contributing new findings in the areas of head injury, hydrocephalus, spinal injury, and achondroplasia. The Neurosurgery faculty provided weekly lectures for medical students with programs for undergraduate medical students, residents, and fellows. Senior medical students had the option of taking a one-month elective in Neurosurgery, while General Surgery junior-level residents rotated through the neurosurgical service on one-month rotations. Fellows in Trauma and clinical fellows took anywhere from six months to one year training in the field.

The Division increased its clinical and laboratory research projects and sought outside funding to support these activities. Dr. Michael E.

Miner, Division Director during much of Moody's tenure as department chair, encouraged research in the department and led the way with his work in trauma-related studies. He also led a team of doctors on visits to Ecuador and Peru where, for several years, they presented lectures and performed surgery on children with severe craniofacial anomalies. The Division hosted an annual conference on neurotrauma for several years that focused on issues including care of the brain-injured patient, from acute care through rehabilitation.[4]

In 1987, the Division expanded its capabilities when John B. Berry, MD, and Hatem S. Megahed, MD, joined the faculty. Berry was interested in identifying patients with cerebrovascular disease who would benefit from surgery and began working with the Department of Neurology to develop a Seizure Surgery Service that would bring together resources to provide better treatment for these patients. Dr. Megahed began working with Hermann Hospital to create an intermediate care unit that would improve the overall efficiency of care. In 1988, the Division and Hermann Hospital opened a twelve-bed Neuro Critical Care Unit (NCCU) with Dr. Hatem Megahed as Medical Director. Other clinical research continued, including a study of children with head injuries, and several studies supported by NIH funding.[5]

The work with Hermann Hospital in time led to the development of a separate department. Funding from the Vivian L. Smith Foundation helped establish the Vivian L. Smith Department of Neurosurgery at The University of Texas Medical School–Houston. With extensive access to complex neurosurgical cases at Memorial Hermann Hospital and in the Texas Medical Center, the new department was created to provide patients with exceptional neurosurgical care and to establish leadership in neurosurgery research and in training new neurosurgeons. In 2005, the Walter M. and Mary A. Mischer Foundation provided funding to launch the Mischer Neuroscience Institute (MNI) at Memorial Hermann–TMC. The Mischer family created the foundation in 1998, as a way to give back to the community in which Walter Mischer Sr. had achieved great success in real estate and business ventures. Since its beginnings, the Mischer Foundation has supported local charities, community projects, and several institutions in the Texas Medical Center (TMC), including UTHealth and M. D. Anderson Cancer Center. The Mischer Neuroscience Institute, with 140 beds and five operating rooms, provides specialized treatment for patients with diseases of the brain and spine. The Institute, a collaborative effort between The University of Texas Medical School–Houston and Memorial Hermann–TMC, is an example of the new team approach to medicine and surgery, with its fully integrated program bringing together neurology, neurosurgery, neuroradiology, and neurorehabilitation into a comprehensive neurological and neurosurgical program.[6]

Orthopaedic Surgery

The Orthopaedic Training Program at The University of Texas Health Science Center in Houston had its origins in Hermann Hospital years before the UT Medical School opened and could rightfully claim to be among the oldest programs in Texas. Taylor K. Smith, MD, served as director of the Division from 1978 through 1984. By the late 1980s, the Orthopaedic Surgery program matured to where it offered residents the opportunity to participate in a number of rotations through affiliated institutions including Hermann, Ben Taub, and St. Joseph hospitals, where they experienced training in "management of musculoskeletal injuries connected with polytrauma, isolated injuries, and fractures of osteoporosis." Residents trained in hand and microvascular surgery, arthroscopy of the knee and shoulder, total joint replacement, surgery of the foot, and general orthopedics, and at M. D. Anderson, they learned to diagnose and manage musculoskeletal tumors. Clinical faculty also served on staff at the Orthopedic Trauma Service at Hermann Hospital and supervised foot, sports medicine, and spine specialty clinics at Hermann and Shriner's hospitals. The full-time faculty included surgeons with subspecialties in spine, general orthopedics, pediatric orthopedics, orthopedic traumatology, post-traumatic reconstruction, infection management, sports medicine, hand and microsurgery, and arthroscopy.[7] After formally becoming a separate department, Orthopaedic Surgery, presently led by Walter R. Lowe, MD, who received his medical degree at the Medical School in 1983, continued to grow and has become a national leader in education, research, and clinical practice. The department continues to offer opportunities for medical students, residents, and fellows at the state's busiest Level I Trauma Center at Memorial Hermann–TMC, and through its Sports Medicine and outreach programs at sixteen clinics in the greater Houston area.[8]

Otorhinolaryngology

During this period, Head and Neck Surgery (ENT—ear, nose, and throat) formed the Department of Otorhinolaryngology. Here the faculty provides clinical care for patients with complex diseases and disorders of the ears, nose, and throat. In addition to the clinical service, the Department also sponsors a residency in otolaryngology and fellowships in facial plastic surgery and rhinology. Physicians from the department also perform research in clinical and basic science projects. The Department's full-time faculty provides subspecialty expertise in a variety of areas within the field of Ear, Nose, and Throat under the direction of Dr. Martin J. Citardi.[9]

Cardiothoracic and Vascular Surgery

The Division of Thoracic and Cardiovascular Surgery, as it was known in the early days of the department, faced unusual challenges from the very beginning. When Stan Dudrick began building the Department of Surgery in 1972, the Texas Medical Center already had two of the leading cardiovascular programs led by two of the most renowned heart surgeons of the twentieth century, Dr. Denton A. Cooley, at the Texas Heart Institute (THI) in St. Luke's Episcopal Hospital, and Dr. Michael E. DeBakey at Baylor College of Medicine and Methodist Hospital. Consequently, students who sought careers in heart surgery preferred to train in those programs and, as a result, despite the best efforts of faculty and long-time division chief, Dr. O. H. "Bud" Frazier, the division languished, much to the consternation of administrators at Hermann Hospital, who understood how profitable heart surgery could be for them.

Dr. Cooley earned his bachelor's degree at The University of Texas in Austin and had attended UTMB for two years of his medical training prior to transferring to Johns Hopkins. His loyalty to UT then made it easy for the Medical School to establish relations with him and the Texas

Heart Institute. This affiliation was beneficial to both institutions and later offered a unique opportunity for participation by the Department of Surgery's organ transplant program. Students at the Medical School who were interested in heart surgery jumped at the opportunity to train under Denton Cooley at THI. The situation had not changed appreciably by Frank Moody's tenure as department chair. "Cardiac Surgery was a problem, because it just wanted to limp along and be part of the Texas Heart Institute, which was fine," said Moody years later. "I worked very closely with Bud Frazier to have a combined program, but cases always were going out to the Texas Heart Institute, which is understandable. It had a reputation. It had Denton Cooley and others." Moody felt the pressure, however, from Hermann Hospital. "The hospital people were always beating up on me, saying, 'How come you don't have more cardiac?'" Moody recalled. "I said, 'Well, we are trying to build it' but I did not solve that problem."[10]

It should be noted that during the 1970s, Cooley donated funds to create the Denton A. Cooley Professorship at The University of Texas Medical School at Houston. Dr. R. Lee Clark, director of The University of Texas M. D. Anderson Cancer Center, lobbied university regents to support converting the professorship into an endowed chair in the Department of Surgery. "I just thought that chair would be one of the best ways of connecting and repaying my debt to The University of Texas," Cooley recalled years later. "I always thought that I had a debt to The University of Texas for giving me such an inexpensive education, and I wanted to repay, in some way, my gratitude to the University for what they had done for me. Dr. Lee Clark convinced the Board of Regents to raise the level to a chair rather than a professorship." Both Frank Moody and later Richard Andrassy would hold the Denton A. Cooley, MD, Chair in Surgery.[11]

Throughout its history, then, the Division of Thoracic and Cardiovascular Surgery has had several chairs, but the surgeon most associated with that role was Dr. Bud Frazier. Frazier, who grew up in Stephenville, Texas, graduated from The University of Texas in 1963 and went to medical school at Baylor College of Medicine, where four years later he received his medical degree. Subsequently, he served as a flight surgeon and assault helicopter medic in the US Army's 48th Assault Helicopter Company in Vietnam (1968–1970) and was awarded the Combat Flight Medal, the Vietnamese Navy Medal, and the Vietnamese Distinguished Service Medal. After his military service, he returned to Houston and completed specialty training in general surgery under Dr. Michael E. DeBakey and Dr. Stanley Crawford at Baylor and then accepted a residency in thoracic and cardiovascular surgery under Dr. Denton A. Cooley at the Texas Heart Institute. Subsequently, Frazier went on to become a pioneer in heart transplantation and in developing artificial devices that assist or could replace functions of the human heart.[12]

Frazier recalled that in the early days of the UT Medical School, Michael DeBakey and Denton Cooley basically had monopolized most of the heart surgery in the Texas Medical Center. The Medical School then focused on hyperalimentation and emergency trauma care, specialties of Drs. Dudrick and Duke, and began working closely with M. D. Anderson for cancer surgery with Dr. Ted Copeland. As Frazier recalled, "[At] UT, they did not even do heart surgery then. But they were going to have emergency care, and they were going to see heart attacks, so they had to have some sort of [cardiac] program. So, even though they did not want to particularly, they started a program." In 1977, Stan Dudrick recruited E. Ross Kyger III, MD, whom he had known at Pennsylvania, and who at that time was Attending Surgeon at the Texas Heart Institute. "He was actually the first person to be involved with any cardiac surgery over there," said Frazier. Kyger had worked with Denton Cooley at Texas Heart Institute and was Attending Surgeon there, 1974–1978. He joined the faculty at the Medical School (1977–1978) and served as Chief of Thoracic and Cardiovascular Surgery at Hermann Hospital until 1978, when he left to go into private practice. "Ross started doing a few heart cases, emergencies for people that could not be transferred to St. Luke's or Methodist," said Frazier. "Nobody wanted to be operated on over there [Hermann Hospital], because they had no reputation or experience. It was always hard to get much of a program, because they were right next door to the biggest [cardiology] programs in the world."[13]

For a time during the 1980s, Dr. William Walker served as division chief, but when he left on a sabbatical in 1987 the department again called on Bud Frazier. "His departure threw me back over there because, again, they did not have anybody," said Frazier. "And so, I was again Chief of Cardiac Surgery but, you know, it was just me. There wasn't anybody else." Frazier recalled how the division struggled to get patients but remembered the role of Drs. Barry Kahan and Charles Van Buren in helping THI implement the use of cyclosporine successfully in heart transplant procedures. "I was interested in transplant particularly as a vehicle for the LVAD [Left Ventricular Assist Device]. So, I came back over here. I was mainly working here [St Luke's]. There was nothing to do over there [Hermann]. They did not do any heart surgery short of emergencies. So, my main activity was here and I was also on the staff at Anderson. I did a lot of work over there." As described earlier, Kahan was instrumental in building up a world-class Division of Immunology and Organ Transplantation. He was one of the leading researchers in the use of immunosuppressant drugs, primarily with kidney transplants. "We did the first heart transplant with cyclosporine on July 4, 1982, and the patient lived ten years," said Frazier. "We would not have been able to start that without Barry Kahan and Chuck Van Buren and cyclosporine, and the serendipity of me being at UT instead of Baylor."[14]

Through the 1980s and into the 1990s, the Division of Thoracic and Cardiovascular Surgery struggled to develop a clinical practice. Since the Texas Heart Institute had the second largest transplant program in the United States, most students with an interest in cardiovascular surgery and most heart patients preferred to be at THI—in Denton Cooley's program—rather than at Hermann Hospital, and thus the UT program mostly languished. Administrators at Hermann Hospital attempted to attract more cardiac transplantation and also more patients for treatment of heart disease. The Division of Thoracic and Cardiovascular Surgery welcomed Dr. Michael S. Sweeney in 1988. Sweeney was well known to Frazier. He received his medical degree at Johns Hopkins and trained at THI before going to the University of South Florida, where he became Chief of Cardiac Surgery and initiated a heart transplant program. But in time, Sweeney realized that he was not too enamored with south Florida. Frazier recollected that Sweeney assisted with transplants at THI and did one of the first transplants at Hermann Hospital. "I cannot remember why we did it at Hermann," said Frazier. "And Sweeney did it and I think I helped, but Sweeney did everything." Eventually, Dr. Sweeney also left to go into private practice. "And then, again, we had a long period where we just really did not have much coverage," said Frazier. In an effort to expand its clinical service, Hermann Hospital developed a second cardiac catheterization laboratory and completed two new cardiovascular operating suites in 1989.[15]

Despite some hopeful signs along the way, then, the cardiovascular service at Hermann Hospital did not attract many patients, and the Medical School's Division of Thoracic and Cardiovascular Surgery remained moribund. On July 1, 1997, however, the first signs of change appeared when Hermann Hospital and Memorial Healthcare System announced a merger. Completed in November, the merger was beneficial to both institutions in that Hermann would be receiving referrals from the much larger Memorial system and Memorial gained both a presence in the Texas Medical Center and a prestigious affiliation with The University of Texas Medical School at Houston.

The board of the new healthcare system immediately set out to make its mark. One area they wanted to enhance was the cardiovascular surgery program at Hermann Hospital. Working in concert, Memorial Hermann and the Medical School began efforts to bring new life to the program and began a search for new leadership in Cardiothoracic and Vascular Surgery. Barely one year after the completion of the merger, on November 8, 1998, officials from those institutions approached Dr. Hazim J. Safi at Baylor College of Medicine in an attempt to recruit him to UT. But Safi was happy where he was as Chief of the Vascular Division at Baylor and at Methodist Hospital, and was not interested in making what was tantamount to a lateral move to UT and Hermann Hospital. Safi proposed that if UT and its Department of Surgery agreed to create a separate new department that would include Thoracic, Cardiac, and Vascular surgery, he would be interested in making the move. Serious negotiations began in December and culminated the following May when The University of Texas, Memorial Hermann Hospital, and Hazim Safi agreed to terms. On September 10, 1999, Dr. Hazim J. Safi began work as Professor and Chair of the new Department of Cardiothoracic and Vascular Surgery. "CV Surgery was part of my department," said Dr. Andrassy. "We were trying to grow it with Hermann Hospital and we were fortunate enough to get Dr. Hazim Safi to come over from Baylor and Methodist where he was a protégé of Dr. DeBakey. As part of the deal of bringing him over, we broke that off as a department." And as Bud Frazier noted later, "Hazim Safi was a very good heart surgeon at that time ... and once Hazim came, then the whole game changed."[16]

Hazim J. Safi, MD grew up in Iraq and first met Dr. Michael DeBakey at a conference in Baghdad during December 1974. A young medical student at the time, Safi was assigned to chauffeur DeBakey around while he was in Baghdad, and the two had time to become acquainted. As he recalled years later, "When I took him to the airport, he said 'We will get you in Houston.' And I waited a year and a half and nothing happened." He was about to travel to England to take a fellowship at the Royal College of Surgeons of England when he finally received a letter from DeBakey. The letter had been misaddressed to "Hazim J. Safi, Baghdad Medical City, Baghdad College of Medicine, Baghdad/India" and sent in December 1974, shortly after DeBakey returned to Houston. "So it took a year and a half to go from India to Iraq in 1976," said Safi. "That is how I came [to Houston]. I am very grateful to the postal office in India to figure out where Baghdad was." Safi trained at Baylor under Dr. DeBakey and Dr. Ernest Stanley Crawford, a highly renowned heart surgeon and one of the pioneers in aortic surgery. Safi remained at Baylor for the next twenty-three years and rose to Professor and Chief of Division of Vascular Surgery.[17]

When Safi made the move to UT in 1999, he brought with him the Chief of the Division of Research, Dr. Charles C. Miller, and most of his team from Baylor, including one vascular surgeon and one cardiac surgeon. Safi had built up a large practice, and his patients soon followed him to UT and to Memorial Hermann Hospital. But he recalled a grueling schedule in which he did nearly 700 cases. "It was tremendous for the hospital, but I could not go home," he recalled. The hospital had not yet constructed its Heart and Vascular Institute, and Safi found himself working in less than ideal conditions. "I was promised operating rooms, four operating rooms, in May 2000," stated Safi. "The operating room I operated in was built in 1946. The beds barely passed through . . . because the [ORs] are built for hernia, hemorrhoids, and stomach operations. Well, we did cardiac, thoracic—which had a lot of other paraphernalia—for quite a while. [But] we survived." In March 2008, the Memorial Hermann Heart & Vascular Institute opened next door to the original Hermann Hospital building. The 230,000 square-foot, freestanding heart and vascular hospital was the first of its kind in the Texas Medical Center and proclaimed itself to be "the most modern hospital of its kind in Texas." The facility has 147 patient beds, including a twenty-bed short stay unit, a Cardiovascular ICU cardiology care unit, and six cardiac catheterization and electrophysiology labs. Within three years after it opened (2010–2011), Memorial Hermann–TMC was recognized as one of the top fifty hospitals for heart and heart surgery by *U.S. News & World Report*.[18]

In addition to its work at the Memorial Hermann Heart & Vascular Institute, the UT Department of Cardiothoracic and Vascular Surgery grew into a very robust department of sixteen surgeons providing services to Memorial Hermann's Southeast and Northeast hospitals and at St. Joseph's Hospital in downtown Houston. The department also became known nationally and internationally as a leader in repairing aortic aneurysms—no surprise, considering Dr. Safi's background. As he observed, "I worked with Dr. Stanley Crawford, who was the guru of aneurysm, and Dr. Michael DeBakey who was considered the one who established vascular surgery and aortic surgery in the world." The department also continues to conduct research and is an active presenter at regional, national, and international conferences. Today, UT students have a wide range of opportunities to learn all aspects of cardiothoracic and vascular surgery and to gain practical experience at both the Texas Heart Institute and the Memorial Hermann Heart and Vascular Institute.[19]

Pediatric Surgery

The most recent of the surgical divisions to convert to full departmental status is Pediatric Surgery. The development of the division under Drs. Richard Andrassy and Kevin Lally is discussed earlier, but it is important to note in this context the rise of the UT Medical School's latest surgical department and the reasons for its new status. Here a changing relationship with the primary teaching hospital, Children's Memorial Hermann, and the rise of new surgical technology with its consequent increase in subspecialization both played a key role.

As noted earlier, Dr. Kevin P. Lally, chair of the department of Pediatric Surgery, first joined the Medical School as faculty in September 1991 and later became division chief when Rich Andrassy was appointed permanent Chair of Surgery in 1995. Lally and Andrassy had a vision to build Pediatric Surgery into one of the best academic pediatric surgical programs in the United States. Their plan was to bring into the division certain surgical specialties that would be able to work as a multi-disciplinary team within the division. Over the years, they continued to move towards that goal even as Memorial Hermann and its children's hospital kept growing. But at the UT medical school, the administrative turnover and the turmoil of the 1990s had faculty wondering what would happen next. Still, by 1999, the division of Pediatric General Surgery included several general surgeons, neurosurgery, plastic surgery, and urology—specialists who could operate on pediatric patients. This vision of a multi-specialty pediatric surgical division ran head on into the financial challenges of the era. As Lally later recalled, "that concept was an important one, [but] it started to fade because the organizational structure did not support it at the time. We had all these subspecialty surgeons related to these other departments, but they were also in the Department of Surgery and in a division of that department. In retrospect, it just was not the right structure to make that happen. But we kept growing in terms of clinical volume."[20]

Meanwhile, Children's Memorial Hermann Hospital continued growing, but the operating room environment remained very adult-oriented. In addition, surgeons had grown weary of dealing with administrative issues that overflowed into the operating rooms, and funding became increasingly problematic. In Texas over half of the children are covered by Medicaid, but Medicaid reimbursement for surgeons remained low, putting a stranglehold on the key revenue stream for the division. Pediatric Surgery is a high-expense endeavor but under Medicaid reimbursement a relatively low income-producing program. This dependence on the state for much of its funding made it difficult to support a full team of pediatric surgical specialists. Consequently, chairs in other departments increasingly had little interest in expanding into the pediatric surgery program and having their specialists participate. "It became apparent that the school's ability to support the subspecialists with the standard financial relationship did not exist," said Lally. "The Medical School's primary mission is research and education, not pediatric subspecialty surgery. So, I don't fault the Medical School, but that was the case." As a result of all this and the growing friction with administrators at the hospital, surgeons were leaving. And because of the growing dissatisfaction, it began to appear that the hospital soon would be grossly understaffed in surgery. In 2003, Memorial Hermann appointed Craig Cordola as Assistant Vice President of Operations for its Children's Hospital. Cordola brought a fresh new approach to the hospital's administration; a hopeful sign to the hospital's surgeons. The following year, he was named CEO of Children's Memorial Hermann Hospital.[21]

Cordola moved to find a remedy for the issues concerning the pediatric surgery service, and the situation slowly began to show signs of improvement. Late in 2006, Cordola, Lally, and officials at the medical school began discussions about creating a new relationship between the two entities. Their proposed plan would pull pediatric surgical subspecialists into one entity—a new academic department—which the Children's Hospital agreed to assist financially. In return, the hospital expected the pediatric surgery service to increase its productivity. The University of Texas Board of Regents approved the agreement, and in September 2007, the Division of Pediatric General Surgery became a separate new department with Dr. Kevin Lally as chair. The new department moved quickly to include or recruit surgeons who specialized in pediatric neurosurgery, congenital heart surgery, and plastic surgery. The plan was to eventually have specialists from other surgical specialties also working with pediatric surgery in a collaboration designed to provide the best, state-of-the-art surgical care for children and also to foster interdisciplinary, collaborative research across divisions and departments in the medical school. Key to these academic affiliations and partnerships was maintaining a close relationship with the Department of Surgery. "And for all intents and purposes, while on paper we changed to a separate department, practically speaking, we very much view ourselves as an integral part of that department as well, and that is the vision for these different divisions too."[22]

Creating the new department of Pediatric Surgery helped improve relations with Memorial Hermann and its Children's Hospital. It also led to formally establishing the position of Surgeon-in-Chief at the Children's Hospital, a leadership position that the hospital would support financially. "That was part of this arrangement as well," said Lally. "I took over that role, a role I had for fifteen years, but it was only a title." Lally noted that the project remains very much a work in progress. "It is a long-term vision," said Lally. "We have a very tightly integrated relationship at the hospital. They cannot survive without us and we cannot either, and to me, it has been apparent for a number of years." Lally viewed his role as surgeon-in-chief and as a university chair as an opportunity to build a strong academic program across the spectrum of pediatric specialties. The new organizational structure and the resulting resolution of distracting issues now allows the department to focus on recent advances in medicine and surgical technology that hold tremendous promise for pediatric surgery. Advances in anesthesia have been critical and enable new surgical procedures on babies. Minimal-access surgery technology has advanced in the last decade and developed special downsized equipment, because the adult-sized devices were too big for use on infants. All of this places the Department of Pediatric Surgery on the edge of a new frontier in patient care, education, and research. Lally noted the effects of change over time: "As we have expanded this hospital and as we have expanded this department and these programs over the last twenty years, my scope of practice has actually decreased, because the really old-school pediatric general surgeon which I trained as did a lot of different things. And now, we are starting to get these dedicated specialists in pediatric and it is a whole different field. It also leads to better expertise and people who really are focused on much more niche areas for children's surgery, so it has been good." The division that started off with Richard Andrassy by himself in 1985 as one, lone pediatric general surgeon now stands as a thriving academic department with eight pediatric general surgeons and a fellowship training program.

Much has changed in the Department of Surgery in the forty-plus years since it first opened in 1972. Whether it was the development of expensive, new technology, the changing dynamics of twenty-first century health care in the United States, or a vision of creating new academic departments as a better way to proceed into the future as an organization, all have had an impact on the Medical School's academic surgery programs. The Department of Surgery at The University of Texas Medical School at Houston has withstood the challenges, adapted to the changes, and stands poised to continue fulfilling its noble mission of producing outstanding surgeons, meeting its commitment to provide outstanding patient care, and leading the way in innovative research.

EPILOGUE

Continuing a Noble Mission

To Produce Outstanding Surgeons

Throughout the decades since 1970, when The University of Texas Board of Regents first appointed Cheves M. Smythe as founding dean of its new medical school in Houston, UT-Houston has grown from an initial enrollment of nineteen students to the sixth-largest medical school in the country. In this nearly half-century of serving the people of Texas, the medical school has weathered the storms, both literal and figurative, that history has thrown against it and continued its mission "to provide the highest quality of education and training of future physicians for the state of Texas."[1] This being Houston, some of those challenges included surviving tropical storms and hurricanes that over the years have wreaked destruction and physically transformed the school. In 1976, storms that flooded the Texas Medical Center also damaged the newly constructed main medical school building and delayed its opening by several months. Tropical Storm Allison in 2001 left billions of dollars in damage in the Houston area, including the destruction of many ground-floor UT laboratories and the loss of laboratory animals and priceless medical research. Hurricane Ike in 2008 damaged the John H. Freeman Building to the extent that officials decided it was more cost-effective to tear it down. Today, a magnificent, new, six-story Medical School Expansion/Research Building rises into the sky where the two-story Freeman Building once stood as the original home for UT-Houston. Learning from the painful lessons of previous floods, a new vivarium is located not in the traditional basement setting but on the top two floors of the Research Building and safely out of reach from any future flood waters. The building is connected to the 875,362 square-foot Main Medical School Building, which in turn connects directly to Memorial Hermann–TMC Hospital.

The Medical School is one of six schools that comprise UTHealth that also includes: the School of Biomedical Informatics, the Dental Branch, the School of Public Health, the School of Nursing, and the Graduate School of Biomedical Sciences. Physician faculty provide the majority of their outpatient care in the UT Professional Building (formerly the Hermann Professional Building), located across the street from the Medical School, and also at a growing number of UT Physicians clinics around the greater Houston area. Since its inception, more than 5,000 physicians have earned their medical degrees at UT-Houston. In addition, the Medical School also provides residency and fellow training as well as continuing education programs for practicing physicians.[2]

In the years since Drs. Stanley J. Dudrick, James H. Duke, Edward M. Copeland, and Senior Resident Dr. Bruce V. MacFadyen first arrived to launch the new Department of Surgery at The University of Texas Medical School–Houston, the department likewise has continued in its mission "to produce outstanding surgeons." During its history, departmental leadership and faculty have consistently demonstrated a willingness to embrace and adapt to change as they sought innovative and better ways to train new surgeons and to provide the best in patient care. In addition, the research conducted in the department has been one of the fundamental pillars on which it has grown. Stan Dudrick brought his pioneering work in Total Parenteral Nutrition (TPN) and attracted colleagues who found new applications for the concept of providing nutrition intravenously to desperately ill patients so they could survive the rigors of surgery. Dudrick and Dr. Red Duke, along with Hermann Hospital's Dan Kadrovach and others, supported the idea of a helicopter ambulance, and Life Flight was born, bringing Houston into a new era in the forefront of trauma care and research. In reflecting on some of the milestones in the department's history, Department Chair Richard J. Andrassy observed that, "Life Flight obviously played an important role in giving Memorial Hermann and UT a lot of publicity to grow into the largest trauma center in America. Dr. Duke and Dr. Dudrick and their innovations made a big contribution to where we were heading." Andrassy noted that lessons learned about air evacuation of casualties and advancements in treating wounded soldiers during the Vietnam War and later conflicts inspired new innovations in trauma care. In addition to its ability to rapidly trans-

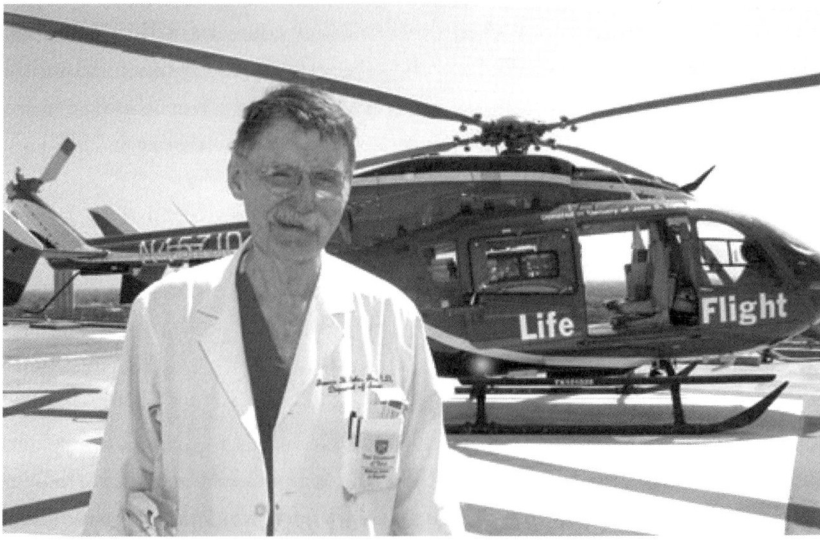

Dr. Red Duke at Life Flight, Memorial Hermann-TMC.

port critically injured patients to Memorial Hermann Trauma Center, Life Flight also carries children with critical neonatal problems from distant hospitals and quickly delivers them to the specialists at the neighboring Children's Memorial Hermann for lifesaving care.

During the early 1980s, Dr. Joseph N. Corriere Jr. provided steady leadership during the search and transition to a new chair, Dr. Frank G. Moody. The Moody era was characterized by a strong emphasis on research, including groundbreaking work and a major role in testing immunosuppressant drugs for organ transplantation led by Dr. Barry Kahan. "I think that organ transplantation has had a big role in the surgery department because of the development of immunosuppressant drugs," said Andrassy. "The early work that Dr. Kahan did in that area, followed by Dr. Charles Van Buren and now by Dr. Bynon, has allowed us to have very active liver transplant, kidney, and heart programs." Administratively, although there had been some movement by a few of the surgical divisions to form separate departments during Stan Dudrick's tenure as chair, this idea began to gain more momentum later and was one of the issues with which Frank Moody had to contend. In addition to dealing with these administrative concerns, Moody supported initial research into laparoscopic surgery and was a pioneer in developing a strong bariatric surgery practice as well.

When Frank Moody announced that he would step down as chair in 1994, the Dean of the Medical School, Dr. John C. Ribble, asked Richard J. Andrassy to fill in on an interim basis while a search committee sought out a permanent chairman. Andrassy quickly proved to be the right person for the position, however, and was appointed on a permanent basis in 1995. Today, nearly twenty years later, Andrassy stands as the longest serving surgery chairman in the country. Under Andrassy, the Department of Surgery continued to lead the way in the areas of minimally invasive surgery, robotics, and pediatric surgery. Andrassy led an era of surgical innovation and administrative changes that introduced a new division, Acute Care Surgery, and a new concept in caring for emergency and trauma cases. Under his watch, the new departments of Pediatric Surgery and Cardiothoracic and Vascular surgery opened. Today, the Department of Surgery is comprised of seven divisions including: Acute Care Surgery, Elective General Surgery, General Surgery/LBJ, Immunology & Organ Transplantation, Oral & Maxillofacial Surgery, Plastic & Reconstructive Surgery, and Urology. Andrassy is Professor and Chairman of the Department and holds the Denton A. Cooley, MD, Chair in Surgery and the Jack H. Mayfield, MD, Distinguished University Chair in Surgery. In considering the many changes in the department during his tenure as chairman, Andrassy observed, "Even though we have broken off into departments, we have grown in areas that did not exist before I took over as chairman. We did not have robotics and we did not have minimally invasive surgery. We did not have many of the areas that we have now, focusing on emergency general surgery and the new resuscitative methods."[3]

Indeed, much has changed from the time Drs. Harold Bailey and George McDonald became the first General Surgery graduates in 1973. By June 2015, the department had provided graduate training for 209 surgeons who graduated from UT-Houston. As discussed throughout the text, many of them have gone on to become pioneers in their specialties and leaders in American surgery, achieving great success in both private practice and in academics. Several alumni shared reflections on their time at UT-Houston in a voluntary survey conducted for this study. Debra

A. Reilly, MD, FACS, presently is Associate Professor, Section of Plastic and Reconstructive Surgery at the University of Nebraska Medical Center. She was at the Medical School from 1983 to1989, and recalled her greatest challenge. "Although I was not the first woman resident, it was still a difficult and physically intense program for women." Her training enabled her to receive a burn fellowship. "Thanks to my training at UT, that fellowship has opened *all* of my subsequent surgical doors for me." Timothy A. Dernbach, MD, presently serves as Director of Vascular Surgery, St. Vincent Health Care in Billings, Montana. Dernbach was one of the first surgical residents, from 1973 to 1979. He recalled that his greatest challenge at the time was "trying to get enough time to eat and sleep!" He appreciated his time at the Medical School and noted, "It was a small program in 1972 and we spent a lot of one-on-one time with our professors, especially Dr. Dudrick and Dr. Duke. We were family!" Christopher W. Conner MD, Specialist, Mohs Surgery and Plastic Surgery, The Woodlands Skincare Surgery Center, The Woodlands, Texas, was at the Medical School from 1975 to 1978 and recalled that time as being very special. "We were a band of brothers. We all lived, ate, and breathed surgery twenty-four hours a day. Recall that there were *no limits* on hours back then." A more recent graduate from the Department of Surgery is Johnny Perez, MD, PhD, Director, Thibodaux Regional Medical Center Weight Management Program, Thibodaux, Louisiana, who was at the Medical School from 1994 to 2002. He saw his greatest challenge during his years as a resident as "learning to make my way in a large academic center with multiple characters (professors) while maintaining my humanity and sense of humor." Perez stated that his training at the Medical School shaped his career in that "the wide breadth of clinical experience gave me the confidence to pursue a full-spectrum, general surgery practice."[4]

Because of the high degree of success achieved by so many graduates of UT-Houston and specifically by its Department of Surgery, administrators anticipate receiving approximately 1,100 applications for just seven residency slots in surgery, not only from Texas but from around the country and internationally. The department will interview about 100 applicants before narrowing the list and making the final selections.[5]

Students and residents in the surgery program at UT-Houston enter a program that is on the leading edge in research and clinical care, but also one that is built upon a proud history and rich tradition of striving for excellence and adapting to change. In writing a history of an institution as dynamic as the Department of Surgery, one finds in the notion of "change over time" a vehicle by which to look back over its history at how the department met its challenges, how it adjusted to change brought by historical forces of the day, and how it might anticipate, cautiously, what the future may hold. Renowned heart surgeon Dr. Denton A. Cooley reflected on changes in surgery during his career. "When I returned to Houston in 1951, a good portion of the surgery was done by people we considered general practitioners, in that they were not board certified and board certification had not been required for hospital staff privileges," said Cooley. "At St. Luke's Hospital when it opened, I think the chief of surgery was a general practitioner, by definition anyway." Cooley believed that the introduction of Baylor College of Medicine into this city and the arrival in 1948 of Dr. Michael E. DeBakey as Head of Surgery had an impact on the profession in Houston. He also noted other changes in surgery over the years. "In the good old days, we always thought that all of us in specialty training had had enough exposure into general surgery," he recalled. "I used to do all sorts of things, from colon surgery to gallbladders and hernias. But then I gradually concerned myself [mainly with] cardiovascular. But . . . we used to joke about it . . . if someone came to me and said, 'Who is the best hernia surgeon in Houston?' I said, 'Do you want the name of the second best?'" Cooley, who was one of the earliest pioneers in heart transplantation, recalled that of the first dozen heart transplants he performed, none of the patients survived more than about fifteen months due to tissue rejection. But, now, thanks to the development of the anti-rejection or immunosuppressant drugs like those pioneered by Dr. Barry Kahan, patients are able to live longer, more normal lives. "And now, you see these guys who are fifteen or twenty years after organ transplant, even cardiac transplantation, who are still healthy and enjoying life," observed Cooley. "There is just a remarkable change over those years, and I do not know what we will do in the future. We might even find some other ways of making tissue compatibility."[6]

Similar to Cooley's experiences, Richard Andrassy pointed to the trend toward increasing specialization in surgery as one of the most dynamic influences in recent years. "When I came out initially, I might do a pediatric hernia one day and an aortic aneurysm the next day and a colon the next day and a thyroid that afternoon," he recalled. "And now, even though you finish all this training and you go through the basics, in a big place like this, what you wind up doing is a whole lot of a couple operations, so you really develop your skills." Andrassy observed that now he focuses primarily on a narrow range of operations and leaves other types of surgery to the specialists in those areas. "The nature of practice has really changed," he stated. "It is not like the old days. Back in the 1960s and 1970s, Dr. Cooley would operate on your heart and then take your gallbladder out and maybe fix your thyroid tomorrow. In these past forty years, the amount of change is just unbelievable. The department and the things that we do are so much different than what we were asked to do years ago, so you really have to keep reinventing yourself as medicine reinvents itself." He also noted that surgery in general has changed from a basically open, more radical procedure to more physiologically based, noninvasive, or minimally invasive techniques. It is rare that today's surgical residents would do any of the cases that he did while in training forty years ago. For example, one of the most common operations residents performed in training was gastric surgery. Stomach surgery for ulcers was common, but essentially it does not exist today because of all the new drugs used to treat those conditions. And the development of modern chemotherapeutic agents has reduced the number of radical procedures and amputations for malignant tumors. Bruce MacFadyen noted, "Over the past years, just in the last ten years, the changes we have seen in the management of breast cancer have been unbelievable. The minimal-access surgery has been a major breakthrough, going from the open cases to the laparoscopy. And certainly, the capabilities of the computer have allowed these things to really develop, with better data and more accurate data collection."[7]

Other areas of change have affected the department as well and generally in a positive way. As discussed earlier, at the time the Medical School opened, many viewed Hermann Hospital as an institution that in some aspects had lost its way. Often, patients viewed it as a charity hospital but were confused by the fact that it was not a true county hospital nor was it a typical private hospital, and thus they preferred to utilize St. Luke's or Methodist hospitals for their surgical care. Today, as one of the Medical School's primary teaching hospitals, Memorial Hermann–TMC is viewed in a more positive light, and as part of the Memorial Hermann Healthcare System, it has become a place that people want to go to for quality care. Today, Memorial Hermann Hospital–TMC is the busiest trauma center in the country and one of the premier hospitals for many different surgical procedures including neurosurgery, orthopedic surgery, cardiac surgery, and mainline areas such as ENT. Memorial Hermann–TMC and Children's Memorial Hermann together offer lifelong care, from the birth of a patient to mid-life care issues including procedures like knee replacements, heart and vascular surgery and organ transplantation, all the way to end-of-life care for dementia and Parkinson's disease. Perceptions of the Medical School have changed over time as well. "When I started practice, there was this feeling that if you were at the medical school, you were over there just teaching and taking care of poor people," said Richard Andrassy. Therefore, patients preferred to go to a private doctor. Today, patients have many options for healthcare but, as Andrassy noted, patients with serious health issues recognize the expertise found at the Medical School. "If you want something done, if you are in Katy, Texas, and you are going to have your brain operated on or something serious, you may want to come down here."[8]

Technology and new regulations also have had an impact on medical schools in general and on The University of Texas Medical School at Houston too. Because of American Council for Graduate Medical Education (ACGME) restrictions on how many hours residents can work—eighty hours per week, effective nationally July 1, 2003—the nature of both teaching and patient care has changed significantly too. Faculty now take on more responsibility for what once was the purview and training ground for residents, with the result that it is now faculty who generally work the longer hours.[9] But, as Andrassy noted, "This whole concept of the eighty-hour work week was never studied scientifically. It was just an emotional thing." Thus the debate over residents' work hours continues, regarding what constitutes the best policy to provide the optimum training experience while reducing the effects of resident fatigue and its impact on patient outcomes. Toward this end, UT-Houston and Memorial Hermann–TMC are participating in a new study, the "Flexibility In Duty Hour Requirements for Surgical Trainees Trial" (FIRST Trial). The FIRST Trial is sponsored and jointly funded by the American Board of Surgery (ABS), the American College of Surgeons (ACS), and the Accreditation Council for Graduate Medical Education (ACGME). Participants for this study will include all ACGME-approved surgical residency programs affiliated with hospitals that participate in the American College of Surgeons National Surgical Quality Improvement Program (ACS NSQIP). Memorial Hermann–TMC is one of 152 hospitals across the country that has elected to participate in the FIRST Trial. The purpose of the study is to determine whether more flexible work hour requirements create any difference in postoperative outcomes compared to the current resident work hours requirements. Interestingly, this one-year study is the first randomized trial using clinically abstracted data to compare the effects of two alternative resident duty hour protocols on patient outcomes. Sponsors anticipate that the study will provide high-quality data that can be used to determine future resident duty hour requirement decisions. The study has randomized different departments around the country to have more flexible hours compared with the present, strict work-hour requirement. "Some of the residents felt that they were not getting an adequate training," stated Andrassy. "They are up all night admitting patients, and then when the patient goes to the OR in the morning, they cannot stay and see the surgery, because their hours are up. [Now] they will be allowed to do that for educational purposes, not just work purposes."[10]

Residents are acutely aware of rapidly developing new technology and generally want opportunities for more training, particularly in their subspecialties. "They feel that they have had limited exposure to certain things, and they want to be more focused in a specialized area," said Andrassy. "If you look at what is happening in practice now, it is really becoming more and more focused and technical—technology-driven—and you cannot do it all. You cannot even keep up with all literature or go to all the meetings." New technology, including smart phones, smart pads, and wide access to knowledge previously found only in libraries, has changed the nature of teaching and learning in medical schools and has brought changes to clinical care as well. Dr. Bruce V. MacFadyen, the first senior resident in the Department of Surgery in 1972, observed the incredible changes in medical education brought about by computers. He noted that when he was an intern, the professors assigned readings from articles located in medical journals in the library and realized the quandary that arose when students discovered the article had been torn out of the journal by some earlier miscreant. "That was all you had—articles in the library," said MacFadyen. "Now, [with the Internet] all these articles are available to everybody. And now, you can go out on the floor seeing patients and you have a problem that comes up, within ten minutes or so, someone has searched the web and found the answer to the very problem you are dealing with. That was never possible before."[11]

Advances in technology not only have an impact on surgery and patient care, but also on how students learn and professors teach. Students today are less interested in sitting through long lectures, especially when they can view presentations on their own via the Internet. Interactive training and use of simulators is gaining prominence. "In the last few years, we finally have begun really pushing on simulators," said Andrassy. "I think that having our surgical residents and medical students practice with simulation and labs and getting facile doing that before they go to the OR with you makes a big difference. Even though we have decreased or compressed the time they have, I think we will be more efficient in the educational part of it, because they will have already been doing this on their own." Dr. Erik B. Wilson concurred and noted that to remain in the forefront with innovation, practicing on simulators also helped reduce problems with experimental surgical procedures. "I think if you are going to do [research] like we do, you really need to have low complications or you cannot justify being an innovator," stated Wilson. "There is so much simulation in practice and lab work that we can do, that you can do really innovative procedures very safely if you have your head and your heart in the right place. And so, it is a different world than when we started doing heart transplants and every heart transplant patient died, or liver transplants and every liver transplant patient died." But Andrassy cautions that with all the emphasis on innovation and technology, it is important to remember the human side of surgery as well. "I think one of the things we are going to have to reevaluate as we push more and more towards technology, towards robots, and towards computers, is to remember our business is still one of compassion and empathy and dealing with the patient," said Andrassy. "And so, I do not know the answer to that, except you just try to continue to work on instilling it in your residents. I think overall, where the department is going—innovation, technology, more specialization, and a more unified, team approach—I think that also we somehow have got to take time along the way for compassion."[12]

Changes will continue in surgery as well. As discussed earlier, the day of the solo practice surgeon is fading into the past, in part due to the administrative responsibilities of maintaining electronic medical records and all the various compliance issues with which today's surgeons must contend. Hospitals are changing too, in that surgery continues to evolve into more of a team approach. When a patient goes to the OR, there is an entire team, ideally working efficiently and in concert, including the surgeon, scrub nurse, circulator, and anesthetist, to provide the best care and quick recovery in the most cost-effective manner. Specialists from different but related disciplines like cardiology and cardiac surgeons, neurosurgery and neurology, pediatric specialties and pediatric surgery, and internal medicine and general surgery are beginning to integrate more and more into teams. Cost effectiveness and the rapid growth of technology are acting as outside forces that may bring down many of the artificial silos of academic medicine—the departments and divisions. Although there always will be a need for general surgeons, today many specialists in surgery and related fields are integrating into teams that all know a little bit about the case to put the patient care together in a more efficient package. It is possible that in the future, medicine likely will demand a team approach due to the continuing advances in science and research into genomics. "I think the biggest thing we are going to see as a change is instead of one operation fitting a whole lot of patients, we are going to find very personalized medical care based on the individual's genetic structure, their cellular structure," said Andrassy. "Patients are going to have a very selective, individualized treatment, more like personal medicine, based on their genomic structure and on their biological response. And a lot of that is going to be driven by computer-generated research into your genetic structure." Andrassy also sees a time where new computer programs and better imaging technology will make it easier to find and identify tumors earlier, leading to less radical surgeries and treatments. Bruce MacFadyen anticipates a wider use of nanotechnology (manipulating properties and miniscule structures at the nanoscale). "I think we are still a ways from that, but I think [medicine] is getting down there at the cellular level," said MacFadyen. "And how the surgeons will be involved with that is going to be for the next generation to figure out. But that will be fun to see how it happens and it is going to happen. There are a lot of issues, so I do not want to be too simplistic. I think it is going to be down to the cellular level, and when surgery can move that way, I think we are going to be doing less and less surgery over time, but it is going to be a transition."[13]

Given the amazing changes in surgery during the past forty years, what does the future hold for the department? It is impossible to predict everything, of course, but with ongoing work in the laboratories and new discoveries already on the horizon, today's surgeons are optimistic and enthusiastic about the future of the department and their profession. With its long heritage of innovation and research, the Department of Surgery has a guide to the future that should keep it in the forefront of all the new surgical technology and changes ahead. "I guess looking at what the future of this department would be, I think we are going to have to keep questioning and innovating, and I think the innovation will be to better and better equipment, and better ways of preventing complications and acquired infections," said Andrassy. "I think we have been fortunate, if you look back, that we have had some innovators like Dr. Dudrick when he started, with total parenteral nutrition. Certainly, Frank Moody was an early advocate of bariatric surgery. He did bariatric surgery before that was cool." Andrassy envisions a department that will carry on this tradition of innovation long after he retires. While he entertains some specific expectations, he also remains the consummate professor and trusts the residents and faculty of the future will find their own creative new ways. "I think that would be a good thing in this big Medical Center to be able to then concentrate on a division of surgical innovation. And what does that mean? I don't know. I think it will mean that all these young people will get together and work it out."[14]

It is that confidence, along with dedication, compassion, and a spirit of camaraderie, that have been hallmarks of the UT-Houston Department of Surgery throughout the years, a lasting legacy on which to build

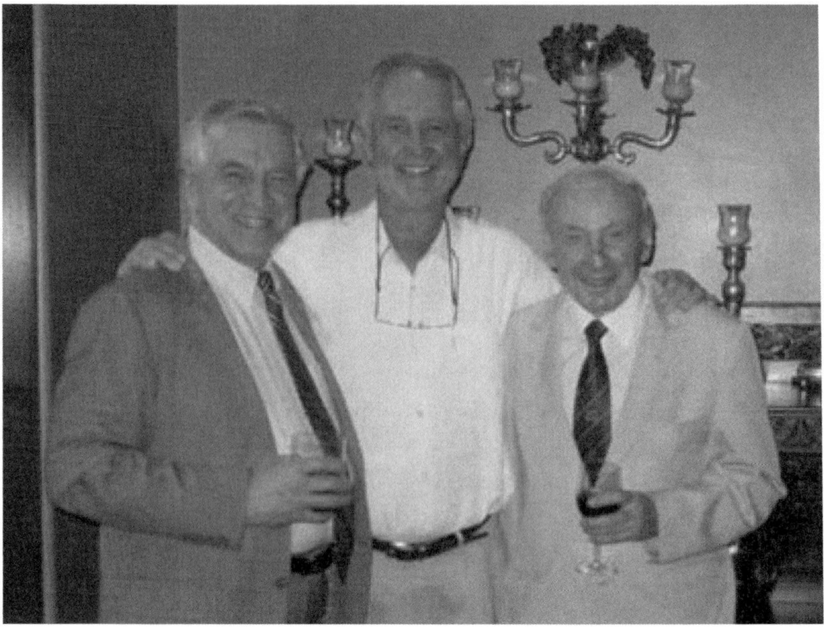

The Three Chairs of the Department of Surgery, L to R: Drs. Stanley J. Dudrick, Richard J. Andrassy, and Frank G. Moody

in the future. Dr. Gilbert A. Castro, a retired UTMS Physiology professor who worked on joint research with some of the surgeons in the early days, recalled how that spirit infused the department of surgery from the beginning. "You can see the gold mine that we had here with Dudrick, Duke, and Copeland and that whole team of surgeons," Castro recalled. "It was unlimited what we could do [in research]. And so that is why it flourished and that is why there was that camaraderie and the fun. And it was fun. Surgeons are fun to be with. They can do anything, and they are all positive."[15]

That positive, confident attitude that they can "fix" whatever is damaged or broken in a human body, along with a deeply held love for their profession and a profound sense of awe for the tremendous responsibility of operating on their patients, is something that the department continues to impart to succeeding generations of surgeons. Despite the often long hours, they remain devoted to their calling and eager to help prepare the new surgeons who soon enough will stand in their places. "I am still working today because I like doing it," said Andrassy. "I think it is fun actually being here doing this, because over the years, you see the change. I was just laughing today when I was operating . . . that the medical students with me now are closer in age to my children and grandchildren. I think it is going to be a different but pretty exciting future here for those who are coming up." Dr. John B. Holcomb expressed his sense of appreciation for the role of the surgeon and the opportunity to repair and help people. "The responsibility and the honor to operate on somebody are pretty amazing," said Holcomb. He noted the significance of the level of trust the patient must have for the surgeon, someone who was a complete stranger just minutes before. "I might meet you and examine you for five minutes and say, 'I'm going to take a knife and cut you open and fix you,' and you will say, 'okay.' It still blows me away that people agree to that." Dr. Red Duke, the department's longest serving faculty member, eloquently spoke of his devotion to the profession and his sense of obli-

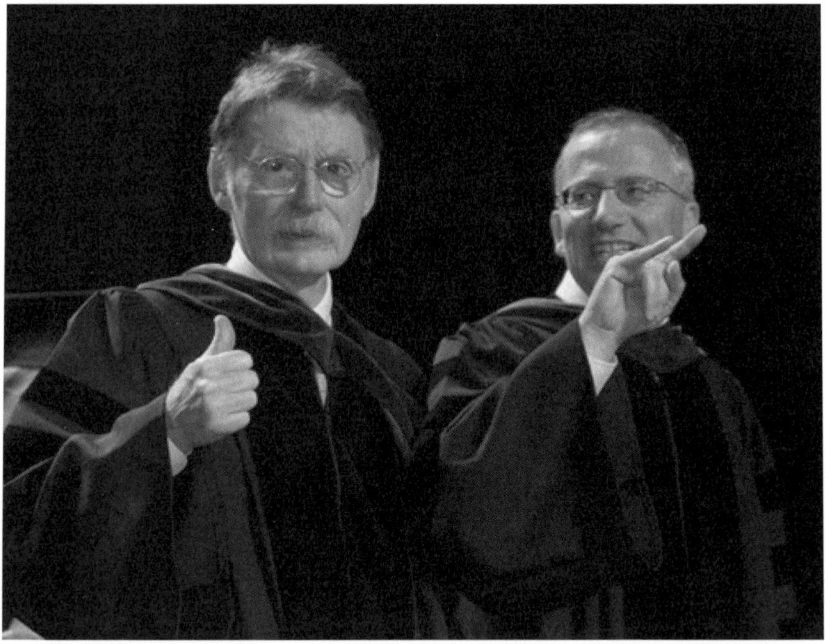

Dr. Red Duke and Giuseppe N. Colasurdo, MD, president, The University of Texas Health Science Center at Houston and dean, The University of Texas Medical School at Houston.

gation to pass along that appreciation to new students. "I really love it," said Duke. "I love taking care of patients. It is such an honor to have the responsibility of being their physician." He noted that for several years administrators asked him to talk to potential students during the recruiting period at the Medical School. "I try to emphasize to them—there is no profession to equal it, because the responsibility is enormous. The privilege of being able to do these things is unspeakable."[16]

After more than forty years of training new surgeons and providing exceptional care for patients in its two teaching hospitals and many satellite clinics, The University of Texas Medical School at Houston Department of Surgery continues its noble mission. The department—its faculty, staff, students, and residents—has survived the many challenges that arose throughout the years and learned to thrive in the highly competitive and richly creative environment of the largest medical complex in the world, the Texas Medical Center. Although it is impossible to predict the future, if its history thus far is any indication, the Department of Surgery will continue to train outstanding surgeons and will stand boldly in the forefront as leaders of innovative research, education, and patient care for many years to come.

APPENDIX

General Surgery Graduates 1973-2015

First Name	Last Name	Degree	Grad Year
Harold	Bailey	M.D.	1973
George	McDonald	M.D.	1973
Bruce	MacFadyen	M.D.	1974
Laurens	Pickard	M.D.	1975
Kenneth	Smith	M.D.	1975
Eduardo	Souchon	M.D.	1976
Michael	Kelly	M.D.	1976
Timothy	Dernbach	M.D.	1977
Stuart	Leventhal	M.D.	1977
Michael	McBee	M.D.	1978
John	Daly	M.D.	1978
Alberto	Maillard	M.D.	1978
Charles	Rodman	M.D.	1978
James	Wallace	M.D.	1978
Susan	Adler	M.D.	1979
Robert	Bloss	M.D.	1979
Albert	Henry	M.D.	1979
David	Ota	M.D.	1979
Charles	Coleman	M.D.	1980
Timothy	Flynn	M.D.	1980
John	Jessup	M.D.	1980
Paul	Pace	M.D.	1980
Alan	Speir	M.D.	1980
Phillip	Adams	M.D.	1981
Laurie	Ahlgren (Latchaw)	M.D.	1981
Ronald	Barton	M.D.	1981
Michael	Hickey	M.D.	1981
Mario	Kapusta	M.D.	1981
Randall	Samberson	M.D.	1981
Thomas	Berry	M.D.	1982

First Name	Last Name	Degree	Grad Year
Ervin	Brown	M.D.	1982
Michael	Carmichael	M.D.	1982
Mark	Gilliland	M.D.	1982
Robert	Hebeler	M.D.	1982
Greg	Pahnke	M.D.	1982
Mary	Brian	M.D.	1983
Christopher	Conner	M.D.	1983
Frances	King	M.D.	1983
Eric	Schaffer	M.D.	1983
John	Stewart	M.D.	1983
Daniel	Bethencourt	M.D.	1984
Eric	Chang-Tung	M.D.	1984
James	Harrell	M.D.	1984
William	Johnson	M.D.	1984
Bruce	Kraemer	M.D.	1984
David	Thompson	M.D.	1984
Ancel	Rogers	M.D.	1985
Alexander	Shadid	M.D.	1985
Lawrence	Sullivan	M.D.	1985
David	Varner	M.D.	1985
Gretchen	Zimmerman	M.D.	1985
David	Corbut	M.D.	1986
Craig	Kuykendall	M.D.	1986
Chris	Malone	M.D.	1986
Richard	Martin	M.D.	1986
Joseph	O'Donnell	M.D.	1986
Wiley	Souba	M.D.	1986
Edson	Cheung	M.D.	1987
Daleela	Jarowenko	M.D.	1987
Timothy	Treece	M.D.	1987
David	Van Buren	M.D.	1987
Richard	Vigness	M.D.	1987

First Name	Last Name	Degree	Grad Year
Edward	Ford	M.D.	1988
Larry	Gentilello	M.D.	1988
Stephen	Hennessey	M.D.	1988
Janet	Hoagland	M.D.	1988
Catherine	Musemeche	M.D.	1988
Basem	Shabb	M.D.	1988
Rolando	Colon	M.D.	1989
Carl	Lagerstrom	M.D.	1989
James	McBath	M.D.	1989
Debra	Reilly	M.D.	1989
Leslie	Cagle	M.D.	1990
Richard	Garza	M.D.	1990
Stuart	Hoff	M.D.	1990
Derrick	McElroy	M.D.	1990
John	Yatsu	M.D.	1990
Michael	Macris	M.D.	1991
Joseph	McIntosh	M.D.	1991
Kelly	Oggero	M.D.	1991
Patrick	Roughneen	M.D.	1991
Brant	Victor	M.D.	1991
Lisa	Florence (Savage)	M.D.	1992
Richard	Hostetter	M.D.	1992
Jason	Nirgiotis	M.D.	1992
Lee	Riley	M.D.	1992
Stephen	Yang	M.D.	1992
Cynthia	Corpron	M.D.	1993
Thomas	Johnston	M.D.	1993
Kimberly	Suppes	M.D.	1993
John	Vega	M.D.	1993
Martin	Beggs	M.D.	1994
Michael	Cortelli	M.D.	1994

First Name	Last Name	Degree	Grad Year
Charles	Cox	M.D.	1994
James	Lonquist	M.D.	1994
Michael	Tornwall	M.D.	1994
Donald	Covington	M.D.	1995
Eric	Munoz	M.D.	1995
Jose	Ortega	M.D.	1995
Paula	Termuhlen	M.D.	1995
Dexter	Turnquest	M.D.	1995
David	Davtyan	M.D.	1996
Pascal	Fuchshuber	M.D.	1996
Rafik	Ghobrial	M.D.	1996
Igor	Gregoric	M.D.	1996
Ruben	Lopez	M.D.	1996
Ara	Vaporciyan	M.D.	1996
Gerardo	Carcamo	M.D.	1997
Philip	Greger	M.D.	1997
Alfredo	Gurmendi	M.D.	1997
John	LoMonaco	M.D.	1997
Charles	Mathis	M.D.	1997
Sadri	Sozer	M.D.	1997
Gary	Allen	M.D.	1998
James	Cross	M.D.	1998
Michael	Hueneke	M.D.	1998
Vijay	Patel	M.D.	1998
Samir	Sukkar	M.D.	1998
Philip	Floyd	M.D.	1999
Eric	Peden	M.D.	1999
Arlene	Ricardo	M.D.	1999
William	Springer	M.D.	1999
Alexandra	Booth	M.D.	2000
Mark	Cockburn	M.D.	2000

First Name	Last Name	Degree	Grad Year
Eileen	Consorti	M.D.	2000
Ming	Pan	M.D.	2000
Emily	Robinson	M.D.	2000
Erik	Beyer	M.D.	2001
Paul	Grant	M.D.	2001
Alicia	Mangram	M.D.	2001
Timothy	Sehorn	M.D.	2001
M. Todd	Wood	M.D.	2001
Antonio	Castaneda	M.D.	2002
Glen	Garner	M.D.	2002
D. Mike	McMullan	M.D.	2002
Holly	Neville	M.D.	2002
Johnny	Perez	M.D.	2002
T. Christopher	Windham	M.D.	2002
David	Ellertson	M.D.	2003
Brijesh	Gill	M.D.	2003
Michael	McBride	M.D.	2003
Galen	Ohnmacht	M.D.	2003
Harvinderpal	Singh	M.D.	2003
Andrew	Harrell	M.D.	2004
Heitham	Hassoun	M.D.	2004
Ganesh	Kumpati	M.D.	2004
Imran	Mohiuddin	M.D.	2004
Joseph	Sucher	M.D.	2004
William	Sumner	M.D.	2004
Erin	Field	M.D.	2005
Christopher	Gullett	M.D.	2005
Johnny	Hong	M.D.	2005
Kelly	Seymour-Dempsey	M.D.	2005
Eduardo	Wolffe	M.D.	2005
Sam	Atallah	M.D.	2006

First Name	Last Name	Degree	Grad Year
Kelly	Gilmore	M.D.	2006
Kenneth	Helmer	M.D.	2006
Steven	Miller	M.D.	2006
Bradley	Putty	M.D.	2006
Sonlee	West	M.D.	2006
Arash	Keyhani	D.O.	2007
Kourosh	Keyhani	D.O.	2007
Donald	Lesslie	D.O.	2007
Stacey	Moore-Olufemi	M.D.	2007
Philip	Rascoe	M.D.	2007
Courtnye Allyson	Walker	M.D.	2007
Michael	Friel	M.D.	2008
Stefanos	Millas	M.D.	2008
James	Suliburk	M.D.	2008
Todd	Wilson	M.D.	2008
Angela	Cheng	M.D.	2009
David	Hamilton	M.D.	2009
Michelle	McNutt	M.D.	2009
Benjamin	Paulson	M.D.	2009
Ravi	Radhakrishnan	M.D.	2009
Thomas (Trey)	Sands	M.D.	2009
Nathan	Allison	M.D.	2010
Christi	Blakkolb	M.D.	2010
Tamara	Ellis	M.D.	2010
Sasha	Kennison-Adams	M.D.	2010
Kenneth	Tieu	M.D.	2010
George	Van Buren	M.D.	2010
Benjamin	Delano	M.D.	2011
Tsuyoshi	Kaneko	M.D.	2011
Erika	Sato	M.D.	2011
Diane	Schwartz	M.D.	2011

First Name	Last Name	Degree	Grad Year
John	Harvin	M.D.	2012
Kenneth	Jastrow	M.D.	2012
Cain	Linville	M.D.	2012
Michelle	Shen	M.D.	2012
Uwe	Fischer	M.D.	2013
Burzeen	Karanjawala	M.D.	2013
Laura	Kreiner	M.D.	2013
Linda	Lesslie	M.D.	2013
Ronak	Patel	D.O.	2013
Shinil	Shah	D.O.	2013
Peter	Walker	M.D.	2013
David	Gochnour	M.D.	2014
Phillip	Letourneau	M.D.	2014
Eric	Sceusi	M.D.	2014
Christopher	Starnes	M.D.	2014
Nicholas	Stephens	M.D.	2014
Allen	Tanner	M.D.	2014
Amit	Agarwal	M.D.	2015
Courtney	El-Zokm	M.D.	2015
Naruhiko	Ikoma	M.D.	2015
Peter	Kneuertz	M.D.	2015
Dhivya	Srinivasa	M.D.	2015
Anthony	Tannous	M.D.	2015

NOTES

Notes to Preface and Acknowledgments

1. Richard Hollingham, *Blood and Guts: A History of Surgery* (New York: St. Martin's Press, 2008) 43-44.
2. Seymour I. Schwartz, MD, *Gifted Hands: America's Most Significant Contributions to Surgery* (New York: Prometheus Books, 2009) 17.

Notes to Introduction

1. The term anatomy, derived from the Greek verb meaning "to cut" or "to dissect," came into being during this time.
2. Wendy Moore, The Knife Man: Blood, Body Snatching, and the Birth of Modern Surgery (New York: Broadway Books, 2005), 66–67.
3. Ibid., 88.
4. Ibid., 22.
5. Irvine Loudon, "Why are (Male) Surgeons Still Addressed as Mr.?" *British Medical Journal*, Vol. 321 (December 23, 2000):1589–1591.
6. Wendy Moore, *The Knife Man*, 69.
7. Ibid., 223; Jeanne E. Abrams, *Revolutionary Medicine: The Founding Fathers and Mothers in Sickness and in Health* (New York: New York University Press, 2013), 101.
8. Atul Gawande, MD, "Two Hundred Years of Surgery," New England Journal of Medicine, Vol. 366 (May 2012): 1716–1723; Jennifer Heisler, RN, "The Evolution of Surgery: A Historical Timeline,"_http://surgery.about.com/od/surgeryinthemedia/a/HistoryOfSurgeryTimeline.html (accessed May 7, 2014).
9. Kenneth Mattox, MD, ed., *The History of Surgery in Houston* (Houston: Houston Surgical Society, 1998), 3.
10. Robert Wooster, "Alexander Wray Ewing," Handbook of Texas Online, http://www.tshaonline.org/handbook/online/articles/few01 (accessed May 14, 2014).
11. Dr. Charles H. McCollum provides a compelling account of the proud civic and medical heritage created by Jones and other early Texas physicians in his introductory essay, "Surgeons and the Texas Revolution," in

Kenneth Mattox, MD, ed., *The History of Surgery in Houston* (Houston: Houston Surgical Society, 1998), 3–15.

12. Inci Bowman, "Beginnings of Medical Journalism in Texas," *Texas Medicine*, 82 (February 1986): 51.
13. Heather Green Wooten, *Old Red: Pioneering Medical Education in Texas* (Denton: Texas State Historical Association Press, 2012), 13–14.
14. Ibid., 3–4; Elizabeth Silverthorne, *Ashbel Smith of Texas* (College Station: Texas A&M University Press, 1982), 218; Watson C. Arnold, "Home Remedies, Folk Medicine, and Mad Stones," *Southwestern Historical Quarterly*, Vol. 117, (No. 2:October 2013):136–137.
15. Chester R. Burns, *Saving Lives, Training Caregivers, Making Discoveries: A Centennial History of The University of Texas Medical Branch at Galveston* (Austin: Texas State Historical Association Press, 2003), 21–22. The anecdote concerning Keiller and his experiments with local anesthesia can be found in *The University of Texas Medical Branch at Galveston: A Seventy-Five year History by the Faculty and Staff* (Austin: University of Texas Press, 1967), 38.
16. D. Clayton Brown, "Medical Education," Handbook of Texas Online http://www.tshaonline.org/handbook/online/articles/sfm02 (accessed May 15, 2014).

Notes to Chapter One

1. On September 25, 1942, The University of Texas Board of Regents formally agreed to name the hospital The M. D. Anderson Hospital for Cancer Research of The University of Texas.
2. Kate Sayen Kirkland, *The Hogg Family and Houston: Philanthropy and the Civic Ideal* (Austin: University of Texas Press, 2009), 60; Frederick C. Elliott, *The Birth of The Texas Medical Center: A Personal Account* (College Station: Texas A&M University Press, 2004) 69–70; Charles LeMaistre, quoted in Bryant Boutwell and John P. McGovern, *Conversation with a Medical School: The University of Texas–Houston Medical School, 1970–2000* (Houston: The University of Texas–Houston Health Science Center, 1999), 4–5. Charles A. LeMaistre, MD, joined the faculty The University of Texas Southwestern Medical School in Dallas in 1959. In 1965, he became Associate Dean of the UT Southwestern Medical School and in 1966 became Vice Chancellor for Health Affairs of The University of Texas System. In 1969, Dr. LeMaistre advanced quickly to Executive Vice Chancellor, then Chancellor-elect and, from

1971 until1978, he served as Chancellor of The University of Texas System. In 1978, he relinquished the position and was appointed President of the M. D. Anderson Cancer Center in Houston, where he served from 1978 to 1996.

3. Kenneth W. Ludmerer, *Time to Heal: American Medical Education from the Turn of the Century to the Era of Managed Care* (Oxford University Press, 1999) 140–142, 210–213; Charles LeMaistre, quoted in Bryant Boutwell and John P. McGovern, *Conversation With a Medical School,* 4–5.
4. L. Rodney Rodgers, MD, "The Birth of The University of Texas Medical School in Houston," *The Good Old Days: Memories of Retired Harris County Physicians,* ed. George Alexander, MD (Austin: Sunbelt Eakin Press, 2001), 146.
5. William S. Fields, MD, *To and Through the Texas Medical Center: A Personal Odyssey* (Austin: Eakin Press, 1995) 246; L. Rodney Rodgers, MD, "The Birth of The University of Texas Medical School in Houston," 151–52.
6. Charles LeMaistre, quoted in Bryant Boutwell and John P. McGovern, *Conversation With a Medical School,* 4–5. Rodgers later wrote about the affiliation agreement between The University of Texas and Hermann Hospital. On November 15, 1967, the hospital's medical staff leaders reviewed the original affiliation agreement at a dinner in the cafeteria. The medical staff agreed with the new structure that included two main committees, the legislative Education Committee and the Medical Board, to replace the hospital's Executive Committee. But the agreement was changed without the knowledge of the medical staff and then signed by HHE trustees and UT regents on January 1, 1968. The altered agreement, which combined the Executive and Education Committees into one Medical Board and gave total control of the medical staff to the School, would lead to a full-scale revolt by doctors at the hospital and a later rebellion by medical school department chairs when officials attempted to update the agreement. See: L. Rodney Rodgers MD., "The Birth of The University of Texas Medical School in Houston," 151–52.
7. Bryant Boutwell and John P. McGovern, *Conversation With a Medical School,* 6–9; L. Rodney Rodgers MD., "The Birth of The University of Texas Medical School in Houston," 153.
8. Cheves M. Smythe, interview by William H. Kellar, March 6, 2012. Cheves M. Smythe, interview by Roberta Hammond, videotape #11 of

The University of Texas Health Science Center Medical School history, March 1995.

9. L. Rodney Rodgers MD., "The Birth of The University of Texas Medical School in Houston, 154–55; Cheves M. Smythe, interview by William H. Kellar, April 13, 2007; Cheves M. Smythe, interview by William H. Kellar, March 6, 2012; Cheves M. Smythe, interview by Roberta Hammond, videotape #11 of The University of Texas Health Science Center Medical School history, March 1995.
10. Cheves M. Smythe, interview by William H. Kellar, April 13, 2007; Cheves M. Smythe, interview by Roberta Hammond, videotape #12 of The University of Texas Health Science Center Medical School history, March 1995.
11. L. Rodney Rodgers MD., "The Birth of The University of Texas Medical School in Houston, 160–61; Cheves M. Smythe, interview by Roberta Hammond, videotape #12 of The University of Texas Health Science Center Medical School history, March 1995; Bryant Boutwell and John P. McGovern, *Conversation With a Medical School,* 13, 24.
12. Cheves M. Smythe, interview by Roberta Hammond, videotape #11 of The University of Texas Health Science Center Medical School history, March 1995; Cheves M. Smythe, interview by William H. Kellar, April 13, 2007.
13. Cheves M. Smythe, interview by William H. Kellar, March 6, 2012; Cheves M. Smythe, interview by Roberta Hammond, videotape #12 of The University of Texas Health Science Center Medical School history, March 1995; Richard Stranahan Ruiz and William Henry Kellar, *Ophthalmology at Hermann Hospital and The University of Texas, Houston: A Personal Perspective* (Houston: Hermann Eye Fund, 2010) 62–67.
14. Cheves M. Smythe, interview by Roberta Hammond, videotape #11 of The University of Texas Health Science Center Medical School history, March 1995; Cheves M. Smythe, interview by William H. Kellar, November 8, 2013; Graeber Obituary, Porter Loring Mortuary Memorial Networks, http://www.porterloring.com/memsol.cgi?user_id=461410, accessed January 3, 2014; "Dr. Philip O'Bryan Montgomery Jr., pathology professor emeritus and UT Southwestern visionary, remembered for his many contributions," *Newsroom,* UT Southwestern Medical Center Website: http://www.utsouthwestern.edu/newsroom/news-releases/year-2006/dr-philip-obryan-montgomery-jr-pathology-professor-emeritus-and-ut-southwestern-visionary-remembered-for-his-many-contributions.html, accessed January 3, 2014; Cheves McCord

Smythe, *An Advantaged Life: Recollections of Cheves McCord Smythe, MD* (Atlanta: Team Forte Inc., 2013) 354–58; 366–67.

15. Cheves M. Smythe, interview by Roberta Hammond, videotapes #11 and #12 of The University of Texas Health Science Center Medical School history, March 1995.
16. Bryant Boutwell, interview by William H. Kellar, March 19, 2013; Cheves M. Smythe, interview by William H. Kellar, April 13, 2007.
17. Cheves M. Smythe, interview by William H. Kellar, March 6, 2012; Cheves M. Smythe, interview by Roberta Hammond, videotape #13 of The University of Texas Health Science Center Medical School history, March 1995. Years later, Smythe ruefully noted, regarding his idea for having programs rather than departments in the Medical School, "I flatly did not succeed in selling that idea, but I think it is still a good idea."
18. Bryant Boutwell and John P. McGovern, *Conversation With a Medical School,* 177–78.
19. Erik Vinnars, MD, PhD, and Douglas Wilmore, MD, "History of Parenteral Nutrition," *Journal of Parenteral and Enteral Nutrition*, Vol. 27, No. 3): 225; Stanley J. Dudrick, MD, "History of Parenteral Nutrition," *Journal of the American College of Nutrition*, Vol. 28, no. 3 (June 2009): 243–51 (esp. 245).
20. Erik Vinnars, MD, and Douglas Wilmore, MD, "History of Parenteral Nutrition,", 225; Penn Surgery Society website: http://surgery.uphs.upenn.edu/?page=history_Rhoads, accessed July 10, 2013.
21. Joseph Corriere, interview by William H. Kellar, September 13, 2012; http://surgery.uphs.upenn.edu/?page=history_Rhoads; Stanley J. Dudrick, MD, "History of Parenteral Nutrition," 243–51 (esp. 243); Douglas W. Wilmore; Stanley J. Dudrick, "Growth and Development of an Infant Receiving All Nutrients Exclusively by Vein," *JAMA*, Vol. 203, no. 10 (1968): 860–64).
22. S. J. Dudrick et al., "Long-Term Parenteral Nutrition with Growth, Development, and Positive Nitrogen Balance," *Surgery* 64 (1968): 134.
23. Seymour I. Schwartz, MD, *Gifted Hands: America's Most Significant Contributions to Surgery* (Amherst, NY: Prometheus Books, 2009), 187–88.
24. Bruce MacFayden interview by William H. Kellar, September 27, 2012; Dudrick, Stanley J; Jonathan E. Rhoads, "New Horizons for Intravenous Feeding," *JAMA*, Vol. 215, no 6 (1971): 939–49; James C. Stevens, "Surgical Nutrition: The Fourth Coming," *JAMA,* Vol. 239, no. 3 (1978): 191–92.

25. Cheves M. Smythe, interview by William H. Kellar, March 6, 2012; Cheves McCord Smythe, *An Advantaged Life,* 400–401.
26. Stanley J. Dudrick, interview by William H. Kellar, April 8, 2013.
27. Ibid.

Notes to Chapter Two

1. Stanley J. Dudrick, interview by William H. Kellar, April 8, 2013.
2. Ibid.
3. Ibid. James IV Association of Surgeons website: http://jamesivassociationsurgeons.com/index.php, accessed August 9, 2013.
4. Stanley J. Dudrick, interview by William H. Kellar, April 8, 2013; Bruce MacFadyen Jr., interview by William H. Kellar, September 27, 2012.
5. James S. Olson, *Making Cancer History: Disease and Discovery at The University of Texas M. D. Anderson Cancer Center* (Baltimore: The Johns Hopkins University Press, 2009), 89. Murray Copeland had been recruited to M. D. Anderson in 1960 by Dr. R. Lee Clark, director of the hospital, to take the position of director of education.
6. Stanley J. Dudrick, interview by William H. Kellar, April 8, 2013; Edward M. Copeland, interview by William H. Kellar, June 5, 2013.
7. James H. "Red" Duke, interview by William H. Kellar, May 22, 2012; Stanley J. Dudrick, interview by William H. Kellar, April 8, 2013; Drew Ware, M. D. "James H. Duke, MD" *The History of Surgery in Houston: Fifty Year Anniversary of the Houston Surgical Society*, ed. Kenneth L. Mattox, MD (Austin: Eakin Press, 1998) 191–93.
8. James H. "Red" Duke, interview by William H. Kellar, May 22, 2012; Stanley J. Dudrick, interview by William H. Kellar, April 8, 2013.
9. Ibid.
10. James H. "Red" Duke, interview by William H. Kellar, May 22, 2012.
11. Bryant Boutwell and John P. McGovern, *Conversation With a Medical School,* 160–63. Construction would begin on Phase II, a 524,000 square-foot structure, the following year.
12. Edward M. Copeland, interview by William H. Kellar, June 5, 2013.
13. Gilbert A. Castro, interview by William H. Kellar, February 6, 2014; Cheves McCord Smythe, *An Advantaged Life,* 357.
14. Stanley J. Dudrick, interview by William H. Kellar, April 8, 2013; Edward M. Copeland, interview by William H. Kellar, June 5, 2013.
15. Stanley J. Dudrick, interview by William H. Kellar, April 8, 2013.
16. Edward M. Copeland, interview by William H. Kellar, June 5, 2013.

17. Stanley J. Dudrick, interview by William H. Kellar, April 8, 2013.
18. Ibid.
19. Ibid.
20. Park Plaza Hospital website: http://www.parkplazahospital.com/en-US/aboutUs/hospitalNews/newsAndArticles/Pages/thehistoryofParkPlaza-Hospital.aspx, accessed August 20, 2013.
21. Stanley J. Dudrick, interviews by William H. Kellar, April 8, 2013 and April 22, 2013.
22. Ibid.; Bruce MacFadyen Jr., interview by William H. Kellar, September 27, 2012.
23. Edward M. Copeland, interview by William H. Kellar, June 5, 2013; Stanley J. Dudrick, interview by William H. Kellar, April 8, 2013.
24. Phillip R. Adams, interview by William H. Kellar, September 13, 2012; Edward M. Copeland, interview by William H. Kellar, June 5, 2013; Kenneth L. Mattox, interview by William H. Kellar, February 7, 2013; Bruce MacFadyen, Jr., interview by William H. Kellar, September 27, 2012.
25. Eduardo Souchon, interview by William H. Kellar, September 5, 2012.
26. Edward M. Copeland, interview by William H. Kellar, June 5, 2013; Stanley J. Dudrick, interview by William H. Kellar, April 22, 2013.
27. Bruce MacFadyen Jr., interview by William H. Kellar, September 27, 2012; Eduardo Souchon, interview by William H. Kellar, September 5, 2012; Dartmouth website: http://www.dartmouth-hitchcock.org/about_dh/wiley_chip_souba_md.html; http://geiselmed.dartmouth.edu/dean/, accessed August 29, 2013.
28. Phillip R. Adams, interview by William H. Kellar, September 13, 2012.
29. Ibid. After two years with Cooley, UT offered Adams a faculty position. Fresh out of training, Adams began his medical practice doing cardiovascular and thoracic surgery at Hermann Hospital and also at St. Luke's with Dr. Cooley. At the same time he was involved with the Department of Surgery and training residents. Adams left Houston briefly to enter a private practice in Tyler, Texas, and then returned to Houston, again in private practice and operating at Hermann Hospital, but not part of the UT department of surgery again until 2010.
30. Ibid.; Bryant Boutwell, interview by William H. Kellar, March 19, 2013; Cheves M. Smythe, interview by William H. Kellar, November 8, 2013; Cheves McCord Smythe, *An Advantaged Life,* 395–96.
31. Eduardo Souchon, interview by William H. Kellar, September 5, 2012.
32. Ibid.

33. Ibid.; Phillip R. Adams, interview by William H. Kellar, September 13, 2012.
34. Cheves M. Smythe, interview by William H. Kellar, March 6, 2012; Cheves McCord Smythe, *An Advantaged Life,* 401.

Notes to Chapter Three

1. http://www.methodisthealth.com/mdhvc.cfm?id=35825; Kenneth L. Mattox, ed., *The History of Surgery in Houston*, 41415.
2. Eduardo Souchon, interview with William H. Kellar, Houston, Texas, September 5, 2012. Two examples: American College of Surgeons' "Resources for the Optimal Care of the Injured Patient," and the 'Advanced Trauma Life Support Course." Kenneth L. Mattox, ed., *The History of Surgery in Houston*, 414-415.)
3. Stanley J. Dudrick, interview by William H. Kellar, April 8, 2013.
4. James H. "Red" Duke, interview by William H. Kellar, May 22, 2012.
5. Stanley J. Dudrick, interview by William H. Kellar, April 8, 2013.
6. Ibid.
7. Ibid.
8. James H. "Red" Duke, interview by William H. Kellar, May 22, 2012; June 5, 2012; Eduardo Souchon, interview by William H. Kellar, September 5, 2012.
9. Stanley J. Dudrick, interview by William H. Kellar, April 8, 2013; Cheves M. Smythe, interview by William H. Kellar, November 8, 2013. See also: Cheves McCord Smythe, *An Advantaged Life,* 390, 404. According to the Memorial Hermann website, Life Flight now completes over 3,000 missions each year and the John S. Dunn Helistop is one of the busiest hospital helistops in the United States. In its thirty-five-year history, Life Flight has flown more than 130,000 patient missions. http://trauma.memorialhermann.org/life-flight/the-history-of-life-flight/, accessed August 30, 2013.
10. Stanley J. Dudrick, interview by William H. Kellar, April 8, 2013.
11. Ibid.
12. James H. "Red" Duke, interview by William H. Kellar, June 5, 2012, St. Anthony Hospital website: http://www.flightforlifecolorado.org/History, accessed August 23, 2013.
13. Stanley J. Dudrick, interview by William H. Kellar, April 8, 2013; James H. "Red" Duke, interview by William H. Kellar, May 22, 2012; June 5, 2012.
14. Stanley J. Dudrick, interview by William H. Kellar, April 8, 2013;

Edward M. Copeland, interview by William H. Kellar, June 5, 2013.

15. Stanley J. Dudrick, interview by William H. Kellar, April 22, 2013; Eduardo Souchon, interview by William H. Kellar, September 5, 2012.
16. James H. "Red" Duke, interview by William H. Kellar, June 5, 2012; Stanley J. Dudrick, interview by William H. Kellar, April 8, 2013.
17. James H. "Red" Duke, interview by William H. Kellar, June 5, 2012; Life Flight website: http://trauma.memorialhermann.org/life-flight/the-history-of-life-flight/, accessed August 30, 2013. Dr. James "Red" Duke continues to serve as Medical Director for Memorial Hermann Life Flight.
18. "Blast, Fire at Texaco Plant Critically Hurt 12," *Houston Chronicle*, March 17, 1977; "Area Hospitals Treating up to 16 Critically Burned in Blast," *Houston Chronicle*, March 18, 1977; "Texaco Blast Probed," *Houston Post*, March 18, 1977.
19. Stanley J. Dudrick, interview by William H. Kellar, April 8, 2013; James H. "Red" Duke, interview by William H. Kellar, June 5, 2012; "Four Refinery Blast Victims Transferred, *Houston Chronicle*, March 19, 1977; "Texaco Accident Kills 5 Workers," *The Evening News*, Newburgh, New York, October 13, 1982; Bush Lewis PLLC website: http://www.bush-lewis.com/_litigation_spanish/results.html#top, accessed September 28, 2013.
20. Stanley J. Dudrick, interview by William H. Kellar, April 8, 2013.
21. Stanley J. Dudrick, interview by William H. Kellar, April 22, 2013; Life Flight website: http://trauma.memorialhermann.org/life-flight/the-history-of-life-flight/, accessed August 30, 2013.
22. Richard J. Andrassy, interview with William H. Kellar, Houston, Texas, April 7, 2012; Frank G. Moody, interview by William H. Kellar, March 14, 2012.
23. John Dunn Foundation website: http://johnsdunnfoundation.org/; Donald H. Parks, interview by William H. Kellar, October 17, 2012. In 1981, the foundation aided a funding drive to save and renovate the Ashbel Smith Building ("Old Red"), the original medical school building of The University of Texas Medical Branch at Galveston.
24. Edward M. Copeland, interview by William H. Kellar, June 5, 2013.
25. Bruce V. MacFadyen Jr., interview by William H. Kellar, September 27, 2012.
26. Ibid.
27. Edward M. Copeland, interview by William H. Kellar, June 5, 2013.
28. Bryan Boutwell and John P. McGovern, *Conversation with a Medical School*, 109.

29. Ibid. http://www.nlm.nih.gov/changingthefaceofmedicine/physicians/biography_44.html
30. Stanley J. Dudrick, interview by William H. Kellar, April 22, 2013.
31. Ibid.
32. Ibid.
33. James H. "Red" Duke, interview by William H. Kellar, June 5, 2012; James H. "Red" Duke, interview by William H. Kellar, May 22, 2012; Drew Ware, "James H. Duke, M. D.," in Kenneth L. Mattox, ed., *The History of Surgery in Houston,* 193–94.
34. Phillip R. Adams, interview by William H. Kellar, September 13, 2012.
35. Stanley J. Dudrick, interview by William H. Kellar, April 22, 2013.

Notes to Chapter Four

1. Bryant Boutwell and John P. McGovern, *Conversation with a Medical School,* 105, 107, 163.
2. Joseph Corriere, interview by William H. Kellar, September 13, 2012.
3. Ibid.; Richard Andrassy, MD, interview by William H. Kellar, April 17, 2012.
4. Stanley J. Dudrick, telephone interview by William H. Kellar, April 22, 2013; Mary Jane Schier, "Surgery Chairman to be Replaced at UT Medical School," *Houston Post,* August 5, 1980, Sec. A, p. 2; "Nicholas C. Chriss, "Doctors, Students Protest UT Firings," *Houston Chronicle,* August 5, 1980, Sec. 1, p. 6; Mary Jane Schier, "Poor Fiscal Management at UT Medical School Alleged, *Houston Post,* August 14, 1980, Sec. A, p. 26; Mary Jane Schier, "UT Surgeons Appeal for Dudrick's Rehiring," *Houston Post,* October 31, 1980; Sec. B, p. 6.
5. Mary Jane Schier, "Top UT System Officials Fly in to Show Support for Health Science Center Chief," *Houston Post,* November 4, 1980, Sec. A, p. 2; "Mary Jane Schier, "Sterling Says All Problems Except Dudrick Issue Resolved," *Houston Post,* November 6, 1980, Sec. A, p.16. Stanley Dudrick, telephone interview by William H. Kellar, April 22, 2013.
6. Frank G. Moody, interview by William H. Kellar, March 14, 2012; Richard Andrassy, interview by William H. Kellar, April 17, 2012.
7. Joseph Corriere, interview by William H. Kellar, September 13, 2012; Ronald Fischer Obituary, http://brown-forward.com/memsol.cgi?user_id=949422
8. Bryant Boutwell and John P. McGovern, *Conversation with a Medical School,* 14; Joseph Corriere, interview by William H. Kellar, September 13, 2012.

9. Seymour L. Schwartz, MD, *Gifted Hands*, 15354.
10. Antoinette C. Ripepi, MD, and Alan T. Cramer, MD, "The Texas Medical Center and the Houston Surgical Society From 1960 to 1970," in Kenneth L. Mattox, MD, ed., *The History of Surgery in Houston*, 34; Denton A. Cooley, MD, *100,000 Hearts: A Surgeon's Memoir* (Austin: Dolph Briscoe Center for American History, The University of Texas at Austin, 2012), 125–43; Seymour L. Schwartz, MD, *Gifted Hands*, 167; Barry D. Kahan, PhD, MD, "Transplantation in Houston," in Kenneth L. Mattox, MD, ed., *The History of Surgery in Houston*, 407–408.
11. Barry D. Kahan, MD "Transplantation in Houston,", 409–10; Eric Berger, "Houston Helped Bring Innovation to Transplants," *Houston Chronicle*, December 23, 2004.
12. Donald G. McNeil, Jr., "Aron Moscona, 87, Biologist Who Explored Embryonic Cells, Dies," *New York Times*, January 25, 2009; "Aaron A. Moscona, PhD, 1921–2009," *UChicagoNews*, (January 26, 2009), http://news.uchicago.edu/article/2009/01/26/aron-moscona-phd-1921-2009, accessed September 19, 2012.
13. Barry D. Kahan, interview by William H. Kellar, May 2, 2013.; Barry Donald Kahan, PhD, MD, "Abbreviated Curriculum Vitae," undated.
14. Joseph Corriere, interview by William H. Kellar, September 13, 2012; Barry D. Kahan, interview by William H. Kellar, May 2, 2013.
15. Marguerite Johnson, "New Library, New Hospital, and A Schism," in *Houston: The Unknown City: 1836–1946* (College Station: Texas A&M University Press, 1991), 249.
16. Bryant Boutwell and John P. McGovern, *Conversation with a Medical School*, 66; Megan Seaholm, "Hermann Hospital," *Handbook of Texas Online*, http://www.tshaonline.org/handbook/online/articles/sbh06, accessed July 15, 2013.
17. Eduardo Souchon, interview by William H. Kellar, September 5, 2012.
18. Joseph Corriere, interview by William H. Kellar, September 13, 2012.
19. Barry D. Kahan, MD "Transplantation in Houston,", 409.
20. Barry D. Kahan, interview by William H. Kellar, May 2, 2013.
21. Charles Van Buren, MD, interview by William H. Kellar, June 18, 2013.
22. Mary Jane Schier, "Missionary Keeps Faith, Gets Kidney Transplant, *Houston Post*, July 1, 1978, Sec. AA-16.
23. "FDA OKs Cyclosporine for Transplants," *American Journal of Nursing*, Vol. 84, No. 1 (January 1984): 9.
24. Barry D. Kahan, interview by William H. Kellar, May 2, 2013; "FDA OKs Cyclosporine for Transplants," 9.

25. Barry D. Kahan, MD "Transplantation in Houston," 410–11; Leslie Gerber, "Extraordinary Program Gives Patients a Chance at Ordinary Lives," http://www.uthouston.edu/distinctions/archive/2007/august/archive.htm?id=876063, accessed May 13, 2013.
26. Charles Van Buren, interview by William H. Kellar, June 18, 2013.
27. Barry D. Kahan, interview by William H. Kellar, May 2, 2013.
28. Charles Van Buren, interview by William H. Kellar, June 18, 2013.
29. Barry D. Kahan, MD, "Transplantation in Houston," 411.
30. Charles Van Buren, interview by William H. Kellar, June 18, 2013.
31. B. D. Kahan, R. H. Kerman, C. A. Wideman, S. M. Flechner, M. Jarowendo, C. T. Van Buren, "Impact of Cyclosporine on Renal Transplant Practice at The University of Texas Medical School at Houston," *American Journal of Kidney Diseases*, Vol. 5, no. 6 (June 1985): 288–95; Eric Berger, "Houston Helped Bring Innovation to Transplants."
32. Barry D. Kahan, interview by William H. Kellar, May 2, 2013.
33. B. D. Kahan, "Fifty Years in the Vineyard of Transplantation: Looking Back," *Transplantation Proceedings*, Vol. 43 (2011): 2853–59; Barry D. Kahan, interview by William H. Kellar, May 2, 2013.
34. Seymour L. Schwartz, MD, *Gifted Hands*, 162–63; "Thomas E. Starzl, MD, PhD," *UPMC: Life Changing Medicine*, http://www.upmc.com/media/experts/Pages/thomas-e-starzl.aspx, accessed August 6, 2013.
35. Rosalind Jackler, "Dual Surprise Greeted Doctors in Liver Surgery," *Houston Post*, July 18, 1976, A-16.
36. Ibid.
37. Charles Van Buren, interview by William H. Kellar, June 18, 2013.
38. Rosalind Jackler, "Dual Surprise Greeted Doctors in Liver Surgery."
39. Seymour L. Schwartz, MD, *Gifted Hands*, 158–59; Rosalind Jackler, "Transplant at Hermann Hospital a Texas First," *Houston Post*, December 9, 1985, A-8.
40. Barry D. Kahan, MD, "Transplantation in Houston,", 411–13; Rosalind Jacker, "Pancreas Patient Improves," *Houston Post*, December 14, 1985, A-17; Charles Van Buren, interview by William H. Kellar, June 18, 2013.
41. Charles Van Buren, interview by William H. Kellar, June 18, 2013.
42. Ibid.
43. Barry D. Kahan, MD, "Transplantation in Houston,", 412; "LifeGift" http://www.lifegift.org/lifegift/info/partners/; "LifeGift" http://www.lifegift.org/lifegift/info/lg_about_us/ ; "Celebrating 25 Years: The Life Gift

Timeline, 1987–2012", http://www.lifegift.org/resources/files/25thAnniversaryTimeLine.pdf.)

Notes to Chapter Five

1. Frank G. Moody, interview by William H. Kellar, February 22, 2012.
2. Ibid.
3. Ibid.
4. Ibid.
5. "Faculty Biography: Frank G. Moody," http://utsurg.uth.tmc.edu/faculty/moody.html
6. Frank G. Moody, interview by William H. Kellar, February 22, 2012.
7. Bryant Boutwell and John P. McGovern, *Conversation with a Medical School*, 33.
8. Bryant Boutwell and John P. McGovern, *Conversation with a Medical School*, 34.
9. Conversation with Ernst Knobil, PhD, in Bryant Boutwell and John P. McGovern, *Conversation with a Medical School*, 37.
10. Frank G. Moody, interview by William H. Kellar, February 22, 2012; Frank G. Moody, MD, *Frank Reflections of an Academic Surgeon* (Bloomington, IN: iUniverse LLC, 2013), 116–17.
11. Bryant Boutwell and John P. McGovern, *Conversation with a Medical School*, 36.
12. Frank G. Moody, interview by William H. Kellar, February 22, 2012.
13. Conversation with Ernst Knobil, PhD, in Bryant Boutwell and John P. McGovern, *Conversation with a Medical School*, 36.
14. Frank G. Moody, interview by William H. Kellar, February 22, 2012.
15. "Faculty Biography: Donald H. Parks, MD," http://utsurg.uth.tmc.edu/faculty/parks.html.
16. Donald H. Parks, interview by William H. Kellar, October 17, 2012.
17. Frank G. Moody, *The University of Texas Medical School at Houston, Department of Surgery Status Report, 1984–1985* (Houston: The University of Texas Medical School, Houston, 1988), 19.
18. Donald H. Parks, interview by William H. Kellar, October 17, 2012.
19. Betsy Paris, *Legacy: 50 Years of loving Care, Texas Children's Hospital, 1954–2004* (Houston: Elisha Freeman Publishing, 2008), 676–77.
20. Ibid., 680.
21. Frank G. Moody, interview by William H. Kellar, March 14, 2012.
22. Ibid.

23. Richard J. Andrassy, interview by William H. Kellar, April 17, 2012.
24. Ibid.
25. Ibid.
26. Bryan Boutwell and John P. McGovern, *Conversation With A Medical School*, 109.
27. Frank G. Moody, *The University of Texas Medical School at Houston, Department of Surgery, Status Report, 1986–1987*, 12–13.
28. Frank G. Moody, *The University of Texas Medical School at Houston, Department of Surgery, Status Report, 1988–1989*, 12.
29. Frank G. Moody, interview by William H. Kellar, March 14, 2012.
30. Ibid.
31. Barry D. Kahan, MD, "Transplantation in Houston,", 411.
32. Bruce V. MacFadyen Jr., MD, "Frank G. Moody, MD," in Kenneth L. Mattox, MD, ed., *The History of Surgery in Houston*, 216.
33. Barry D. Kahan, MD, "Transplantation in Houston,", 411–12.
34. Bruce V. MacFadyen Jr., MD, "Frank G. Moody, MD,", 216.
35. Barry D. Kahan, interview by William H. Kellar, May 2, 2013.
36. Ibid.
37. Bruce MacFadyen Jr., MD, "Frank G. Moody, MD," 215–16.
38. Frank G. Moody, interview by William H. Kellar, February 22, 2012.
39. Ibid.
40. Ibid.
41. Ibid.
42. Ibid.
43. Bruce MacFadyen Jr., MD, "Frank G. Moody, MD," 216.
44. Frank G. Moody, *The University of Texas Medical School at Houston, Department of Surgery, Status Report, 19881989*, 25.
45. Frank G. Moody, interview by William H. Kellar, February 22, 2012.
46. Frank G. Moody, *The University of Texas Medical School at Houston, Department of Surgery, Status Report, 1988–1989*, 25.
47. Frank G. Moody, interview by William H. Kellar, March 14, 2012.
48. Ibid.
49. Ibid.
50. Bruce V. MacFadyen Jr., MD, "Frank G. Moody, MD," 216.
51. Frank G. Moody, interview by William H. Kellar, March 14, 2012.
52. Ibid.
53. Bruce V. MacFadyen Jr., MD, "Frank G. Moody, MD," 218.
54. Frank G. Moody, interview by William H. Kellar, March 14, 2012.
55. Bruce V. MacFadyen Jr., MD, "Frank G. Moody, MD," 218.

56. John C. Ribble, "Standing Ground/Setting Course," in Bryant Boutwell and John P. McGovern, *Conversation with a Medical School*, 52; John C. Ribble, interview by William H. Kellar, February 5, 2013.
57. Frank G. Moody, interview by William H. Kellar, February 22, 2012.
58. Frank G. Moody, MD, *Frank Reflections of an Academic Surgeon* (Bloomington, Indiana: iUniverse, LLC, 2013) 167.
59. Harris Health website: https://www.harrishealth.org/en/about-us/who-we-are/pages/history.aspx, accessed September 22, 2013.
60. John C. Ribble, "Standing Ground/Setting Course,", 52; see also: John C. Ribble, interview by William H. Kellar, February 5, 2013.
61. Frank G. Moody, interview by William H. Kellar, March 14, 2012.
62. Frank G. Moody, interview by William H. Kellar, February 22, 2012.
63. Frank G. Moody, interview by William H. Kellar, March 14, 2012.
64. Eduardo A. Souchon, interview by William H. Kellar, September 5, 2012.
65. Bruce V. MacFadyen Jr., MD, "Frank G. Moody, MD," 218.
66. Richard J. Andrassy, interview by William H. Kellar, April 17, 2012.

Notes to Chapter Six

1. Richard Andrassy, interview by William H. Kellar, December 9, 2013.
2. Richard Andrassy, interview by Kevin Lally, April 2, 2011.
3. Richard Andrassy, interview by William H. Kellar, December 9, 2013.
4. Ibid.
5. Richard Andrassy, interview by William H. Kellar, April 17, 2012.
6. Richard Andrassy, interview by Kevin Lally, April 2, 2011.
7. Richard Andrassy, interview by William H. Kellar, December 9, 2013.
8. Ibid.
9. Ibid. Today, the VMI biology department enjoys a sizable private endowment named in honor of "Doc" Carroll. Supplied through the generosity of loyal VMI alumni, the fund has grown has grown significantly over the years, providing money for equipment purchases and affording the department the opportunity to monetarily reward cadets for outstanding academic performance.
10. Richard Andrassy, interview by Kevin Lally, April 2, 2011.
11. Richard Andrassy, interview by William H. Kellar, December 9, 2013.
12. Richard Andrassy, interview by Kevin Lally, April 2, 2011.
13. "The Battle of New Market," Virginia Military Institute Archives, http://

www.vmi.edu/Archives/Civil_War/New_Market/Battle_of_New_Market_Home/ (accessed January 30, 2014); Charles R. Knight, "Valley Thunder: The Battle of New Market, *Hallowed Ground Magazine* (Summer 2010): http://www.civilwar.org/hallowed-ground-magazine/summer-2010/valley-thunder-battle-of-new-market.html (accessed January 30, 2014).

14. Since 1887, VMI cadets have participated in an annual reenactment of the Battle of New Market, inclusive of a ninety-mile march to the battlefield. However, in recent years, Andrassy noted, most go by bus. Richard Andrassy, interview by William H. Kellar, December 9, 2013.
15. Richard Andrassy, interview by William H. Kellar, December 9, 2013.
16. Richard Andrassy, interview by William H. Kellar, January 7, 2014.
17. Richard Andrassy, interview by William H. Kellar, December 9, 2013. "Major General (Dr.) James William Humphreys," *Biography, United States Air Force* (July 1, 1967), http://www.af.mil/AboutUs/Biographies/Display/tabid/225/Article/106736/major-general-dr-james-william-humphreys-jr.aspx, accessed: January 3, 2014.
18. Richard Andrassy, interview by Kevin Lally, April 2, 2011.
19. "David Hume, MD," Virginia Commonwealth University, http://www.vcuhealth.org/?id=427&sid=1 (Accessed: January 6, 2014; "About Dr. David Hume," http://www.surgery.vcu.edu/humera_new/hume.html, accessed: January 6, 2014.
20. Richard Andrassy, interview by Kevin Lally, April 2, 2011.
21. Richard Andrassy, interview by William H. Kellar, December 9, 2013.
22. Richard Andrassy, interview by Kevin Lally, April 2, 2011.
23. Ibid.
24. Ibid.
25. Ladd's career in pediatric surgery began as a result of a tragic event during World War I. In 1917, two ships—a Norwegian passenger liner and a French cargo vessel loaded with wartime explosives—collided in the harbor of Halifax, Nova Scotia. The accident set off a tremendous explosion that resulted in over 11,000 casualties. As one of the volunteer surgeons who went to Halifax, Ladd cared for many of the injured children on board the SS *Imo*. The sobering experience compelled him to shift gears and devote his career only to pediatric surgery. See: William Hardy Hendren III, MD, "Pediatric Surgery," *Pediatrics*, Vol. 102 (July 1, 1998): 275–78.
26. Betsey Parish, *Legacy: Fifty Years of Loving Care*, 672; http://childrenshospitalblog.org/happy-75th-birthday-congenital-heart-defect-surgery/.

27. William Hardy Hendren III, MD, "Pediatric Surgery," 275; William E. Ladd, MD, "The Surgical Treatment of Esophageal Atresia and Tracheo-esophageal Fistulas," *New England Journal of Medicine*, Vol. 230 (No. 21, May 25, 1944): 625–37; C. Everett Koop, "A Perspective on the Early Days of Pediatric Surgery, " *Journal of Pediatric Surgery*, 33, no. 7 (July 1988); http://www.childrenshospital.org/about-us/our-history-and-innovations/historical-milestones; Betsey Parish, *Legacy: Fifty Years of Loving Care*, 672.
28. Richard Andrassy, interview by William H. Kellar, December 9, 2013; William Hardy Hendren III, MD, "Pediatric Surgery," 275.
29. J. A. Wolff, College of Physicians and Surgeons, Columbia University, "The History of Pediatric Oncology," *Pediatric Hematology and Oncology*, Vol. 8 (April–June, 1991): 82–91; "Biography: Sidney Farmer, MD," http://www.learntoquestion.com/seevak/groups/2007/sites/farber/bio.html, accessed: January 9, 2014.
30. Richard Andrassy, interview by William H. Kellar, December 9, 2013.
31. Richard Andrassy, interview by William H. Kellar, April 17, 2012.
32. Richard Andrassy, interview by Kevin Lally, April 2, 2011.
33. Richard Andrassy, interview by William H. Kellar, December 9, 2013.
34. Ibid.
35. Ibid.
36. Ibid.
37. Kevin Lally, interview by William H. Kellar, September 6, 2012.
38. Ibid.
39. Richard Andrassy, interview by William H. Kellar, April 17, 2012.
40. Ibid.
41. As a ship's surgeon on board the USS *Aulick*, Able sustained multiple severe, lasting injuries when a kamikaze plane blew apart the ship in November 1944. He received the Purple Heart, the Silver Star, and three combat citations for his actions in the Pacific. Kenneth L. Mattox, MD, ed., *The History of Surgery in Houston*, 74–75.
42. Harris County ranked first in the nation for value of industrial construction, and with building permits of $266,802,075 for the country and $100,160,322 for the city, in 1948. "Houston 'Tops' Industrially," *Houston*, XX (April 1949), 24; "Houston Leads Nation in Per Capital Building," *Houston*, XX (April 1949), 8.
43. Between 1946 and 1964, the national birthrate grew by 78 million. *Texas Almanac*, 1966–1967, 135; J. Virgil Scott, "Houston Banks Grow," *Houston*, XV (September 1943), 6; "Houston: Southwest Money

Market," *Houston*, XXXV (October 1964), 63; David G. McComb, *Houston: The Bayou City* (Austin: University of Texas Press, 1969), 189.
44. Luke W. Able, Oral History, June 18, 1979; Betsey Parish, *Legacy: Fifty Years of Loving*, 673.
45. Luke W. Able, Oral History, June 18, 1979; Betsey Parish, *Legacy: Fifty Years of Loving*, 673.
46. Dedicated to babies and children with diagnostic and treatment issues that could not be remedied elsewhere, Texas Children's Hospital has evolved into a 639 licensed-bed, full-care pediatric center boasting an annual count of approximately 20,000 inpatient and over 300,000 outpatient visits. No longer conjoined with St. Luke's Episcopal Hospital, Texas Children's Hospital is central to a defined network of healthcare services that includes Texas Children's Pediatric Associates, Texas Children's Health Centers, Texas Children's Health Plan, and Texas Children's International. Betsey Parish, *Legacy: Fifty Years of Loving Care*, x.
47. Ibid., 95.
48. Ibid., 674.
49. In July 1985, the same month that Andrassy began at UT-Houston, Dr. Bill Pokorny left private practice to join the full-time faculty of Baylor College of Medicine. He became a full professor of pediatric surgery in 1991 and is credited with building from ground up the pediatric surgical division at Baylor. Richard Andrassy, interview by Kevin Lally, April 2, 2011.
50. Richard Andrassy, interview by William H. Kellar, December 9, 2013.
51. Kevin Lally, interview by William H. Kellar, September 6, 2012.
52. Ibid.
53. Richard Andrassy, interview by William H. Kellar, April 17, 2012.
54. Kevin Lally, interview by William H. Kellar, September 6, 2012; Richard Andrassy, interview by Kevin Lally, April 2, 2011.
55. Richard Andrassy, interview by Kevin Lally, April 2, 2011.
56. Richard Andrassy, interview by William H. Kellar, April 17, 2012.
57. Ibid.
58. Ibid.
59. Richard Andrassy, interview by Kevin Lally, April 2, 2011.
60. Richard Andrassy, interview by William H. Kellar, April 17, 2012.
61. Ibid.
62. Richard Andrassy, interview by William H. Kellar, January 7, 2013.
63. Phillip R. Adams, interview by William H. Kellar, September 13, 2012.
64. Richard Andrassy, interview by William H. Kellar, January 7, 2013.

65. In 2011, Moore left the Methodist Hospital in Houston for his current position as Chief of Acute Care Surgery at the University of Florida at Gainesville. "UF Announces New Acute Care Surgery Chief," *Gainesville Sun*, July 7, 2011.
66. Alex Berenson, "Army's Aggressive Surgeon is Too Aggressive For Some," *New York Times*, November 6, 2007; "Distinguished Alumnus Honored by College of Medicine," *University of Arkansas for Medical Sciences*, September 4, 2013, http://www.uamshealth.com/news/?id=5351&sid=1&nid=9930&cid=6 (accessed February 27, 2014); John B. Holcomb interview by William H. Kellar, September 20, 2012.
67. Kevin Lally, Interview by William H. Kellar, September 6, 2012.
68. Children's Memorial Hermann Hospital http://childrens.memorialhermann.org/er/ (accessed February 26, 2014).
69. Kevin Lally, interview by William H. Kellar, September 6, 2012.
70. In 2009, Andrassy was honored along with the Arnold M. Salzberg Award from the American Academy of Pediatrics. The award is given to pediatric surgeons who have distinguished themselves as mentors to pediatric surgical trainees. "2009 AAP Award Winners," American Academy of Pediatrics website: http://aapnews.aappublications.org/content/30/10/27.1.extract#, accessed June 18, 2014; "American Academy of Pediatrics Honors Andrassy," *Scoop*, November 5, 2009, http://med.uth.tmc.edu/comm/Scoop/archive/2009/11/scoop-2009-11-05.html, accessed February 26, 2012.
71. Kevin Lally, interview by William H. Kellar, September 6, 2012.
72. Richard Andrassy, Interview by William H. Kellar, January 7, 2014; Deborah Mann Lake, "Born Inside Out," *Health Leader* (April 18, 2012) http://www.uthealthleader.org/index/article.htm?id=5628c217-b939-439c-a63a-267934bcb7fd (Accessed February 27, 2014).
73. Richard Andrassy, interview by William H. Kellar, January 7, 2014.
74. Deborah Mann Lake, "Born Inside Out," (accessed February 27, 2014).
75. Deborah Mann Lake, "Born Inside Out," (accessed February 27, 2014); Richard Andrassy, interview by Kevin Lally, April 2, 2011.
76. Richard Andrassy, interview by Kevin Lally, April 2, 2011; Deborah Mann Lake, "Born Inside Out," (accessed February 27, 2014).
77. Richard Andrassy, interview by William H. Kellar, January 7, 2014.
78. Richard Andrassy, interview by Kevin Lally, April 2, 2011.
79. Ibid.

Notes to Chapter Seven

1. Frank G. Moody, *The University of Texas Medical School at Houston Department of Surgery Status Report, 1986–87*, 3; Richard J. Andrassy, interview by William H. Kellar, April 9, 2013; April 17, 2012.
2. John B. Holcomb, interview by William H. Kellar, September 20, 2012; United States Special Operations Command, *Task Force Ranger Operations in Somalia, 3–4 October 1993* (United States Special Operations Command, History Offices, 1 June 1994) 1. In late August 1993, Secretary of Defense Les Aspin authorized the deployment of a joint special operations task force (JSOTF) to Mogadishu, Somalia, because of increased enemy attacks on United States and United Nations Operations Somalia (UNOSOM) forces and installations. The special operations forces, named Task Force Ranger, had the mission to capture Gen. Mohammed Farah Aideed and designated others, and to turn over captives to UNOSOM forces. "On October 3, TF Ranger launched a mission into Aideed's stronghold, seeking to capture two of his key lieutenants. The capture of 24 Aideed supporters was accomplished, but in that process, a TF Ranger MH-60 BLACKHAWK helicopter was shot down by a rocket-propelled grenade. The mission then irrevocably changed from one of capturing Aideed supporters to one of safeguarding and recovering American casualties. When the TF Ranger forces finally returned to its compound the next morning, their casualties totaled 99."
3. John B. Holcomb, interview by William H. Kellar, September 20, 2012.
4. Richard J. Andrassy, interview by William H. Kellar, April 17, 2012; John B. Holcomb, interview by William H. Kellar, September 20, 2012.
5. Memorial Hermann–TMC Press Release: "Memorial Hermann–TMC establishes The Texas Trauma Institute," May 29, 2012. Trauma patients also have access to additional services essential to trauma care: trauma and neuro critical care; trauma surgery; orthopedic surgery; emergency general surgery; emergency medicine, neurology and neurosurgery, oral maxillofacial, plastic and ENT surgery; hand surgery and plastic reconstructive surgery; transfusion medicine, physical medicine and rehabilitation; OB/GYN; urology; ophthalmology; heart and vascular; anesthesia; radiology; and hospitalists. Memorial Hermann–TMC Website: http://www.memorialhermann.org/news/memorial-hermann-tmc-establishes-the-texas-trauma-institute/, accessed March 31, 2014.
6. Lora Hines, "Memorial Hermann to Begin Expansion, Renovation at TMC," *Houston Chronicle*, April 16, 2014. http://www.houston-

chronicle.com/business/medical/article/Memorial-Hermann-to-begin-expansion-renovation-5406802.php, accessed April 16, 2014.

7. John B. Holcomb, interview by William H. Kellar, September 20, 2012.
8. Rebecca Heliot, "Police Being Armed with Combat Tourniquets," *Houston Chronicle*, February 6, 2014. http://www.houstonchronicle.com/news/houston-texas/houston/article/Police-being-armed-with-combat-tourniquets-5212730.php?cmpid=hcec, accessed February 8, 2014; John B. Holcomb, interview by William H. Kellar, September 20, 2012.
9. John B. Holcomb, interview by William H. Kellar, September 20, 2012.
10. Ibid.
11. Richard J. Andrassy, interview by William H. Kellar, April 17, 2012; Frank G. Moody, *The University of Texas Medical School at Houston Department of Surgery Status Report, 1984–85* , 13.
12. E. W. D'Anton, *Memories: A History of The University of Texas Dental Branch at Houston* (Houston: The University of Texas Health Science Center at Houston Dental Branch, 1991), 2–3; Frederick C. Elliott, *The Birth of the Texas Medical Center,* 40–41; 126; University of Texas Dental Branch website: http://db.uth.tmc.edu/education/advanced-education-programs/oral-maxillofacial-surgery/program-history, accessed January 21, 2014.
13. Donald H. Parks, interview by William H. Kellar, October 12, 2012. David E. Beesinger, a native of Lubbock, Texas, graduated from Texas Tech University, and he earned a medical degree from The University of Texas Medical School in San Antonio. He served his surgery residency at Parkland Hospital in Dallas and then returned as faculty at Texas Tech Medical School from 1978 to 1979. Following this, Beesinger came to Houston, where he joined Stan Dudrick in the Department of Surgery at the Department of Surgery at The University of Texas Medical School in Houston. He served as director of the Burn Unit at Herman Hospital from 1979 to 1983. *Lubbock Avalanche-Journal,* Obituaries: lubbockonline.com http://lubbockonline.com/stories/061198/042-6146.001.shtml, accessed April 21, 2014. Beesinger died at only fifty-two years of age on June 9, 1998, in Lubbock.
14. Donald H. Parks, interview by William H. Kellar, October 12, 2012.
15. Ibid.; http://trauma.memorialhermann.org/services/burn-treatment-houston/, accessed April 21, 2014.
16. Donald H. Parks, interview by William H. Kellar, October 12, 2012.
17. Ibid.; Camp Janus Website: http://www.campjanus.org/, accessed April 28, 2014.

18. Donald H. Parks, interview by William H. Kellar, October 12, 2012.
19. Ibid.

Notes to Chapter Eight

1. Richard J. Andrassy, interview by William H. Kellar, January 7, 2014. David W. Mercer received his MD in 1986 from the University of Wisconsin–Madison Medical School. He did his internship and then residency and fellowship at Temple University Hospital in Philadelphia. In 1993, he joined the faculty at The University of Texas Medical School at Houston and served as Chief of Surgery at LBJ General Hospital from 1998 to 2006. Today, Dr. Mercer is Professor, Division of General Surgery, McLaughlin Professor and Chairman, Department of Surgery at the University of Nebraska Medical Center. University of Nebraska Medical Center Website: http://www.unmc.edu/surgery/mercer_david.htm, accessed March 11, 2014.
2. Tien C. Ko, interview by William H. Kellar, December 9, 2013.
3. Ibid.; Cheves McCord Smythe, *An Advantaged Life,* 575–79.
4. Tien C. Ko, interview by William H. Kellar, December 9, 2013. Dr. Tien C. Ko was born in Taipei, Taiwan. His family moved to Los Angeles when he was ten. He graduated from UCLA Medical School in 1986 and did his residency at Loyola University Medical Center and then went to UTMB in Galveston to do a research fellowship with Dr. James Thompson. He remained on faculty until February 1, 2007, when he moved to UTMS–Houston and was appointed as Chief of Surgery at Lyndon B. Johnson General Hospital. Presently, Tien C. Ko, MD, is the Jack H. Mayfield Distinguished Professor of Surgery, Vice Chairman for Harris County Hospital District, and Chief of Surgery at Lyndon B. Johnson General Hospital.
5. Tien C. Ko, interview by William H. Kellar, December 9, 2013.
6. Ibid.; Harris Health System website: https://www.harrishealth.org/en/services/locations/pages/lbj.aspx, accessed February 28, 2014.
7. Tien C. Ko, interview by William H. Kellar, December 9, 2013.
8. Eduardo Souchon, interview by William H. Kellar, September 5, 2012; Tien C. Ko, interview by William H. Kellar, December 9, 2013.
9. Jeffrey Ponsky, MD, presently is Chairman, Department of Surgery, University Hospitals Case Medical Center, Professor of Surgery, CWRU School of Medicine, and is Surgeon-in-Chief, University Hospitals.
10. Bruce V. MacFadyen Jr., interview by William H. Kellar, September 27, 2012.

11. Ibid. MacFadyen served as Professor and Chairman of Surgery at Georgia Regents University in Augusta, Georgia. Georgia Regents Health System is a not-for-profit corporation that manages the clinical operations associated with Georgia Regents University. The health system includes the 478-bed Georgia Regents Medical Center; the Georgia Regents Medical Office Building, with more than eighty outpatient practice sites in one convenient setting; the Critical Care Center, housing a thirteen-county regional Level I Trauma Center; the 154-bed Children's Hospital of Georgia; and a variety of centers and units such as the Sports Medicine Center and Georgia Regents Radiation Therapy Center. GR Health website: http://www.grhealth.org/about-us/ContentPage.aspx?nd=364, accessed February 20, 2014.
12. Bruce V. MacFadyen,Jr., interview by William H. Kellar, September 27, 2012; Covidien website: http://www.covidien.com/covidien/pages.aspx?page=AboutUs/Mission, accessed March 3, 2014. Covidien is dedicated to creating and delivering innovative healthcare solutions, developed in ethical collaboration with medical professionals, which enhance the quality of life for patients and improve outcomes for customers. Ethicon Endo-Surgery today is known as Ethicon, and is part of Johnson & Johnson. For more information see: http://www.ethicon.com/corporate, accessed March 3, 2014.
13. Among the leaders in developing endoscopic surgical techniques, MacFadyen cited Dr. George Berci, Senior Director of Minimally Invasive Endoscopic Research at Cedars-Sinai in Los Angeles, who was one of the first people to help develop coherent light transmission. In his forty-plus years at Cedars-Sinai, Berci was a pioneer in the field developing "new visualization techniques, instrument minimizing and high-definition cameras." He was a pioneer in endoscopy techniques and technologies, which later included creating and using an enhanced endoscopic method to intubate patients with particularly difficult airways and video microscopy. Cedars-Sinai Website: http://www.cedars-sinai.edu/About-Us/News/News-Releases-2011-/Cedars-Sinai-Surgeon-George-Berci-Honored-by-American-College-of-Surgeons-for-50-Years-of-Innovations-That-Have-Transformed-Surgery.aspx, accessed March 1, 2014.
14. Erik B. Wilson earned a BS in Science at Texas A&M University in 1992 and graduated from Baylor College of Medicine in 1996. He then did his residency in General Surgery (1996–2000) at Texas A&M University Health Science Center–Scott & White Memorial Hospital, Temple, Texas. From 2000 to 2001, Wilson was General Surgery Administrative

Chief Resident and Clinical Instructor, Texas A&M University Health Science Center–Scott & White Memorial Hospital, Temple, Texas. The following year, 2001–2002, he was a Laparoendoscopic Fellow with Philip L. Leggett, MD, at The University of Texas Health Science Center at Houston.

15. Terry Scarborough is a native of Clovis, New Mexico. Scarborough earned a degree in Pharmacy from the University of New Mexico in Albuquerque. In 1993, Scarborough received his medical degree from the University of New Mexico School of Medicine. He performed his surgery residency at the Baylor College of Medicine in Houston and then completed a year-long fellowship in laparoscopic surgery, also at Baylor. He then joined New Mexico Surgical Associates in Albuquerque and in May of 2000, he performed New Mexico's first laparoscopic kidney transplant. Dr. Scarborough joined The University of Texas Medical School at Houston in 2002, becoming a fellowship director in laparoscopic surgery. Dr. Scarborough joined Dr. Sherman Yu in private practice with Texas Laparoscopic Consultants in June, 2008. Texas Laparoscopic Consultants Website: http://www.tlcsurgery.com/education/program/bariatric-surgeons/dr-scarborough-houston-tx/, accessed March 6, 2014.
16. Erik B. Wilson, interview by William H. Kellar, November 26, 2013. Erik B. Wilson, MD, is Associate Professor of Surgery, Director of the Division of Elective General Surgery and he is also Director of the Minimally Invasive Surgeons of Texas (MIST). See also: Frank G. Moody, MD, *Frank Reflections of an Academic Surgeon*, 184.
17. Erik B. Wilson, interview by William H. Kellar, November 26, 2013; 17 Specialty Surgery Center at: http://www.utphysicians.com/1189/surgery/, accessed March 6, 2014.
18. Erik B. Wilson, interview by William H. Kellar, November 26, 2013.
19. MIST Website: https://med.uth.edu/surgery/education/fellowship/, accessed February 27, 2014. MIST Fellowship Consortium is accredited by the Minimally Invasive Surgery Fellowship Council. Colorectal Surgical Associates Website: http://houstoncolon.com/about/colorectal-surgeon-dr-haas-texas/, accessed March 11, 2014.
20. Erik B. Wilson, interview by William H. Kellar, November 26, 2013.
21. Ibid.
22. Ibid.
23. Ibid.
24. Ibid.

25. Terry Scarborough and Sherman Yu, MD, who trained in the MIST Fellowship and worked for a time at UT, later went into private practice and formed Texas Laparoscopic Consultants. At the time of this writing in 2014, the Division of Elective General Surgery included: Anil Kulkarni, MSC, PhD; Frank G. Moody, MD; Brad E. Snyder, MD; Todd D. Wilson, MD; Emily K. Robinson, MD; Sheilendra Mehta, MD; Donald Lesslie, D.O.; Richard K. Englehardt, MD; Kulvinder S. Bajwa, MD; and Richard J. Andrassy, MD. Division Website: https://med.uth.edu/ surgery/divisions/elective-general-surgery/, accessed March 10, 2014.
26. Joseph N. Corriere Jr., interview by William H. Kellar, September 18, 2012; Baylor College of Medicine website: http://www.larrylipshultz.com/about/dr-larry-lipshultz, accessed April 3, 2014.
27. Joseph N. Corriere Jr., interview by William H. Kellar, September 18, 2012.
28. Vanderbilt University School of Medicine: http://www.mc.vanderbilt.edu/root/vumc.php?site=urologicsurgery &doc=24682
29. Joseph N. Corriere Jr., interview by William H. Kellar, September 18, 2012.
30. Frank G. Moody, *The University of Texas Medical School at Houston Department of Surgery Status Report, 1984–85,* 23. Frank G. Moody, *The University of Texas Medical School at Houston Department of Surgery Status Report, 1986–87,* 19; Frank G. Moody, *The University of Texas Medical School at Houston Department of Surgery Status Report, 1987–88*, 18–19; http://www.webmd.com/kidney-stones/extracorporeal-shock-wave-lithotripsy-eswl-for-kidney-stones, accessed April 21, 2014.
31. Joseph N. Corriere Jr., interview by William H. Kellar, September 18, 2012; Edward J. McGuire, MD, served on the faculty of Yale University (1971–1983), the University of Michigan (1983–1992), and The University of Texas Health Science Center (1992–1999). He returned to the University of Michigan faculty as a professor of urology and head of the Neurourology and Pelvic Reconstructive Surgery Division in 1999, and was named Reed Nesbit Professor of Urology in 2007. An internationally recognized scholar, Dr. McGuire's pioneering work has led to the development of numerous innovative therapies that are now regarded as the standard of care. Edward J. McGuire, MD, Reed Nesbit Professor of Urology and professor of urology in the Medical School, retired from active faculty status on June 30, 2013.
32. Joseph N. Corriere Jr., interview by William H. Kellar, September 18,

2012. Dr. Corriere served as president elect (1992–1993) and then president (1993–1994) of the South Central Section of American Urological Association and as president elect (2004–2005) and president (2005–2006) of the American Urological Association.

33. Joseph N. Corriere Jr., interview by William H. Kellar, September 18, 2012.
34. Richard J. Andrassy, interview by William H. Kellar, April 17, 2012; UT Houston Website: http://www.uth.tmc.edu/urology/, accessed October 21, 2013; http://www.uth.tmc.edu/urology/residents.html, accessed February 20, 2014.
35. Richard J. Andrassy, interview by William H. Kellar, April 17, 2012; http://www.uth.tmc.edu/schools/med/surgery/organ_transplant/index.html, accessed October 21, 2013.

Notes to Chapter Nine

1. Richard J. Andrassy, interview by William H. Kellar, April 9, 2013.
2. Ibid.
3. Frank G. Moody, interview by William H. Kellar, February 22, 2012; Frank G. Moody, *The University of Texas Medical School at Houston Department of Surgery Status Report, 1984–85* , 5.
4. Frank G. Moody, *The University of Texas Medical School at Houston Department of Surgery Status Report, 1986-87*, 6–11.
5. Frank G. Moody, *The University of Texas Medical School at Houston Department of Surgery Status Report, 1987-88* , 6–7; Frank G. Moody, *The University of Texas Medical School at Houston Department of Surgery Status Report, 1988–89* , 6–7.
6. UTMS Website: http://www.uth.tmc.edu/schools/med/neurosurg/, accessed March 25, 2014; Memorial Hermann TMC website: http://neuro.memorialhermann.org/about-the-institute/, accessed October 21, 2013; Mischer website: http://mischer.com/who-we-are/mischer-gives-back, accessed March 22, 2014.
7. Frank G. Moody, *The University of Texas Medical School at Houston Department of Surgery Status Report, 1984–89.* 15; Frank G. Moody, *The University of Texas Medical School at Houston Department of Surgery Status Report, 1986-87* , 11; Frank G. Moody, *The University of Texas Medical School at Houston Department of Surgery Status Report, 1987-88* ,10–11; Frank G. Moody, *The University of Texas Medical School at Houston Department of Surgery Status Report, 1988-89* , 10–11.

8. UTMS Orthopaedic Surgery Website: https://med.uth.edu/ortho/chair-message/, accessed October 21, 2013.
9. UTMS Otorhinolaryngology Website: https://med.uth.edu/orl/, accessed October 21, 2013.
10. Frank G. Moody, interview by William H. Kellar, February 22, 2012.
11. Denton A. Cooley, interview by William H. Kellar, March 20, 2013.
12. O. H. "Bud" Frazier, interview by William H. Kellar, November 12, 2013; THI website: http://www.texasheart.org/PatientCare/O_H_Frazier_MD.cfm, accessed May 27, 2014. Bud Frazier has performed over 1,100 heart transplants and has implanted over 700 Left Ventricular Assist Devices (LVADs).
13. O. H. "Bud" Frazier, interview by William H. Kellar, November 12, 2013. At this writing, Frazier is Chief, Cardiopulmonary Transplantation; Program Director and Chief, Center for Cardiac Support; Director of Cardiovascular Surgery Research, Texas Heart Institute. He also is Chief of Transplant Service at St. Luke's Medical Center. Among his academic appointments, Dr. Frazier is Professor of Surgery, University of Texas Health Science Center in Houston; Clinical Associate Professor of Surgery, University of Texas M. D. Anderson Cancer Center; and tenured professor, Baylor College of Medicine in Houston. THI website: http://www.texasheart.org/ PatientCare/O_H_Frazier_MD.cfm, accessed May 27, 2014. Information on Dr. Kyger from: Houston Chronicle online obituaries: http://www.legacy.com/obituaries/houstonchronicle/obituary.aspx?pid=125495347, accessed May 29, 2014.
14. O. H. "Bud" Frazier, interview by William H. Kellar, November 12, 2013.
15. Frank G. Moody, *The University of Texas Medical School at Houston Department of Surgery Status Report, 1988-89* , 16–17.
16. Hazim J. Safi, interview by William H. Kellar, February 4, 2014; Richard J. Andrassy, interview by William H. Kellar, April 17, 2012; O. H. "Bud" Frazier, interview by William H. Kellar, November 12, 2013.
17. Hazim J. Safi, interview by William H. Kellar, February 4, 2014. At this writing, Dr. Safi is the Chairman of The University of Texas, Department of Cardiothoracic and Vascular Surgery. He is also Chief of Cardiothoracic and Vascular Surgery at Memorial Hermann Heart and Vascular Institute.
18. Hazim J. Safi, interview by William H. Kellar, February 4, 2014; http://heart.memorialhermann.org/locations/about-heart---vascular-insti-

tute-texas-medical-center/, accessed May 31, 2014; https://med.uth.edu/cvs/patient-care/heart-surgery/, accessed March 26, 2014.

19. Hazim J. Safi, interview by William H. Kellar, February 4, 2014.
20. Kevin P. Lally, interview by William H. Kellar, September 6, 2012.
21. Ibid. Children's Memorial Hermann Hospital was founded in 1986 and is the primary teaching hospital for the pediatric and obstetrics/gynecology programs at The University of Texas Medical School at Houston. Children's Memorial Hermann offers care to more than 37,000 children each year. http://childrens.memorialhermann.org/about-us/our-history/, accessed May 29, 2014. After a total of seven years at Children's Memorial Hermann, Craig Cordola was appointed CEO of Memorial Hermann–TMC in 2010.
22. Kevin P. Lally, interview by William H. Kellar, September 6, 2012.

Notes to Epilogue

1. The Mission of The University of Texas Medical School–Houston, is "to provide the highest quality of education and training of future physicians for the state of Texas, in harmony with the state's diverse population; to conduct the highest caliber of research in the biomedical and health sciences; and to provide exemplary clinical services in relationship to our educational and discovery activities." The University of Texas Medical School at Houston website: https://med.uth.edu/about/, accessed June 26, 2014.
2. *UT Health Factbook-2014*: http://www.uthouston.edu/fact-book/school-profiles/medical-school.htm, accessed June 25, 2014. Figures include FY 2013, ending August 2013.
3. Richard J. Andrassy, interview by William H. Kellar, June 17, 2014.
4. Comments from: "The University of Texas Medical School-Houston, Department of Surgery Historical Project—Alumni Questionnaire," Spring 2013.
5. Richard J. Andrassy, interview by William H. Kellar, April 17, 2012.
6. Denton A. Cooley, interview by William H. Kellar, March 20, 2013.
7. Richard J. Andrassy, interview by William H. Kellar, April 17, 2012; Bruce V. MacFadyen Jr., interview by William H. Kellar, September 27, 2012.
8. Richard J. Andrassy, interview by William H. Kellar, June 17, 2014.
9. "Libby Zion Law" adopted by New York in 1989 following the death of Libby Zion in 1984 and subsequent lawsuit blaming overworked med-

ical resident. The American Council for Graduate Medical Education (ACGME) made this a national standard in 2003.

10. The FIRST Trial website: http://www.thefirsttrial.org/, accessed June 28, 2014; Richard J. Andrassy, interview by William H. Kellar, June 17, 2014.
11. Bruce V. MacFadyen Jr., interview by William H. Kellar, September 27, 2012.
12. Erik B. Wilson, interview by William H. Kellar, November 26, 2013; Richard J. Andrassy, interview by William H. Kellar, June 17, 2014.
13. Richard J. Andrassy, interview by William H. Kellar, June 17, 2014; Bruce V. MacFadyen Jr., interview by William H. Kellar, September 27, 2012.
14. Richard J. Andrassy, interview by William H. Kellar, June 17, 2014.
15. Gilbert A. Castro, interview by William H. Kellar, February 6, 2014.
16. Richard J. Andrassy, interview by William H. Kellar, April 17, 2012; June 17, 2014; John B. Holcomb, interview by William H. Kellar, September 20, 2012; James H. "Red" Duke, interview by William H. Kellar, May 22, 2012.

A Note on Sources

The secondary literature used in this study is cited in the endnotes that appear for each chapter. Primary research materials for this history came from several major sources including the University of Texas Medical School–Houston Department of Surgery; the John P. McGovern Historical Collections and Research Center, Houston Academy of Medicine–Texas Medical Center Library; the Houston Metropolitan Research Center, Houston Public Library; and Special Collections of the University of Houston–Clear Lake Alfred R. Neumann Library.

There are several sources for the oral history interviews utilized in this project. First, the interviews conducted 2012–14 by the author, William H. Kellar. In addition, during 1995, Roberta Hammond, University of Texas Health Science Center at Houston, conducted a series of videotaped interviews with the medical school's founding dean, Cheves M. Smythe, and his administrative assistant, Sondra Ives. Finally, in 2011, Dr. Kevin P. Lally interviewed Dr. Richard Andrassy as part of a historical project for the American Academy of Pediatrics.

Interviews Conducted by William H. Kellar

Name	**Date of Interview**
Phillip R. Adams, MD	September 13, 2012
Richard J. Andrassy, MD	April 17, 2012; April 9, 2013; December 9, 2013; June 17, 2014
Bryant Boutwell, DR, PH	March 19, 2013
Gilbert A. Castro, MD	February 6, 2014
Denton A. Cooley, MD	March 20, 2013
Joseph N. Corriere Jr., MD	September 18, 2012
Edward M. "Ted" Copeland, MD	June 5, 2013
Stanley J. Dudrick, MD	April 8, 2013; April 22, 2013

James H. "Red" Duke, MD	May 22, 2012; June 5, 2012; July 17, 2012; August 1, 2012
O. H. "Bud" Frazier, MD	November 12, 2013
John B. Holcomb, MD	September 20, 2012
Barry D. Kahan, MD	May 2, 2013
Tien C. Ko, MD	December 9, 2013
Kevin P. Lally, MD	September 6, 2012
Bruce V. MacFadyen Jr., MD	September 27, 2012
Kenneth L. Mattox, MD	February 7, 2013
Frank G. Moody, MD	February 22, 2012; March 14, 2012; March 28, 2012
Donald H. Parks, MD	October 17, 2012
John C. Ribble, MD	February 5, 2013
Hazim J. Safi, MD	February 3, 2014
Cheves M. Smythe, MD	March 6, 2012, November 8, 2013
Eduardo A. Souchon, MD	September 5, 2012
Charles T. Van Buren, MD	June 18, 2013
Erik B. Wilson, MD	November 26, 2013

UTMS Interviews from Video Tapes—Courtesy: Bryant M. Boutwell

Dr. Cheves M. Smythe by Roberta Hammond (four tapes), March 1995

Sondra Ives by Roberta Hammond (three tapes), March 27, 1995

Richard J. Andrassy by Kevin P. Lally, April 2, 2011

INDEX

Note: Page numbers in *italics* indicate photos; page numbers followed by "*n*" indicate endnotes.